MW00511887

Introduction to Clinical Research in Communication Disorders

INTRODUCTION TO CLINICAL RESEARCH IN COMMUNICATION DISORDERS

MARY H. PANNBACKER, PH.D.
Professor and Director, Communication Disorders
Louisiana State University Medical Center

GRACE F. MIDDLETON, ED.D.
Professor of Speech-Language Pathology
University of Texas at El Paso

WITH CONTRIBUTIONS FROM
DAVID L. IRWIN, NORMAN J. LASS,
ANN S. OWEN, AND WILLIS L. OWEN

SINGULAR PUBLISHING GROUP, INC.
SAN DIEGO, CALIFORNIA

Singular Publishing Group, Inc.
4284 41st Street
San Diego, California 92105-1197

© 1994 by Singular Publishing Group, Inc.

Typeset in 10/12 Times by ExecuStaff
Printed in the United States of America by BookCrafters

Library of Congress Cataloging-in-Publication Data

Pannbacker, Mary H.
    Introduction to clinical research in communication disorders /
Mary H. Pannbacker, Grace F. Middleton.
        p.   cm.
    Includes bibliographical references and index.
    ISBN 1-56593-219-6
    1. Communicative disorders—Research—Statistical methods.
I. Middleton, Grace F.   II. Title.
    [DNLM: 1. Communicative Disorders—epidemiology.   2. Data
Interpretation, Statistical.   3. Research Design.   WM 4785 1984]
RC423.P25   1994
616.85'5'0072—dc20
DNLM/DLC
for Library of Congress   94-8061
                                                                CIP

Contents

TABLES

FIGURES

CONTRIBUTORS

David L. Irwin, Ph.D.
Professor and Head of Department of Communicative Disorders
Northeast Louisiana University
Monroe, Louisiana

Norman J. Lass, Ph.D.
Professor of Speech Pathology and Audiology
University of West Virginia
Morgantown, West Virginia

Grace F. Middleton, Ed.D.
Professor of Speech-Language Pathology
University of Texas at El Paso
El Paso, Texas

Ann S. Owen, Ph.D.
Associate Professor of Communication Sciences and Disorders
University of Oklahoma Health Sciences Center
Oklahoma City, Oklahoma

Willis L. Owen, Ph.D.
Associate Professor of Biostatistics and Epidemiology
University of Oklahoma Health Sciences Center
Oklahoma City, Oklahoma

Mary H. Pannbacker, Ph.D.
Professor and Director, Department of Communication Disorders
Louisiana State University Medical Center
Shreveport, Louisiana

PREFACE

The original impetus for this book arose from the senior editor's attempts to teach a basic survey course in research for master's degree students in speech-language pathology. There was no single textbook that fit the needs of the course, and it was necessary to supplement information from several sources. It was difficult to find texts that provided appropriate coverage of the material especially about research training, mentoring, ethical issues, information sources, research utilization, poster presentations, and writing grant proposals. The only way to fill this void was to write a book about research in communication disorders.

This book is intended for anyone interested in research in communication disorders, including students, clinicians, academicians, and researchers. The purpose of this book is to provide a source of current information that is relevant to clinical research. Practicing clinicians have a special need to be knowledgeable about research because of its importance in diagnosis and treatment of speech-language and hearing problems. The book can be used in classes for advanced undergraduate and graduate students in speech-language pathology and audiology. It also should be of value to practicing professionals in communication disorders and other health-related disciplines.

The book contains 10 chapters. Chapter 1 describes the role of research in communication disorders. Chapter 2 discusses the need for ethical guidelines and ethical issues related to subjects, researchers, editors, consumers of research, authorship, and publication. Chapter 3 contains an overview of research. Chapters 4 and 5 are devoted to research strategies and designs. Chapter 6 deals with organization and analysis of research data. Chapter 7 consists of information about research planning. This is followed by Chapter 8 which contains information about research utilization in communication disorders. Chapter 9 addresses reasons and strategies for reporting research. Chapter 10 provides information about writing grant proposals. Readers who require additional information are referred to sources containing more detailed explanations. Study exercises are included to help readers understand and apply the material.

Several people require special thanks: The four contributors, Norman J. Lass, David L. Irwin, Ann S. Owen, and Willis L. Owen, who shared their expertise and experience in this book, and Lorraine Tubbs who provided most of the illustrations. Two people have typed various portions of this book — Gertha Allen and Betty Lorich. Finally our thanks to our mentors and students from whom we have learned much about research in communication disorders.

Dedication

This book is lovingly dedicated to our parents Eleanor Galbraith Hicks and W. W. Hicks and Elsie Pisell Frederick and J. W. Frederick. They encouraged and inspired us to think for ourselves, make a contribution, and to enjoy life to its fullest. The senior author would also like to express her appreciation to Carl and Mozelle Crouch for their support and encouragement.

C H A P T E R 1

COMMUNICATION DISORDERS AND THE ROLE OF RESEARCH

GRACE F. MIDDLETON

- Importance of Research in Communication Disorders
- Historical Evolution of Research in Communication Disorders
- Future Directions of Research in Communication Disorders
- Summary
- Study Exercises
- Suggested Readings

The vitality and endurance of a profession are dependent on the quantity and quality of its ongoing research programs. The curricula of speech-language pathology programs traditionally have reserved the study of research methods and responsibilities for advanced graduate training. By that time students may have developed an attitude of apprehension about research. Sometimes these attitudes develop into sheer terror. Some academic advisors in programs having a thesis option rather than a thesis requirement have difficulty persuading entering graduate students to consider pursuing a thesis project. By the time the students become informed and confident about doing research, they are so far along in their graduate programs that doing a thesis would delay graduation. The purpose of this text is to remove the mystery surrounding research by teaching basic principles and providing practice in gathering and summarizing data. It is hoped that this information will be conveyed to students early in their training in an effort to increase the number of research projects conducted by speech-language pathology students. Once students have developed research skills under the direction of productive faculty, they are more likely to continue the practice as they move into varied professional settings.

IMPORTANCE OF RESEARCH IN
COMMUNICATION DISORDERS

There are a number of reasons for doing research in communication disorders. Short-term or survival objectives for doing research include doing projects to complete one's education or to improve one's job security in an academic setting where tenure and promotion depend on research productivity. More important reasons for doing research include contributing to the professional pool of knowledge about treatment of clients presenting a variety of communication disorders and maintaining quality clinical services while realizing a sense of professionalism by active involvement in learning through discovery. For the person who enjoys receiving professional recognition (and who doesn't?) along with the opportunity to be creative, satisfy curiosities, and engage in problem solving with a team of colleagues having similar interests, research can provide numerous secondary rewards (Pannbacker & Middleton, 1991–1992).

A profession's image is readily enhanced by the integration of research along with the provision of clinical services. Such a practice increases professionalism, accountability to clients and other professionals, and the social relevance of the health services delivered in an economy with increased costs and decreased resources. Clinical research may be readily integrated into the assessment, planning, intervention, and evaluation phases of clinical management (Polit & Hungler, 1991). Findley and DeLisa (1990) stress the importance of integrating clinical and research activities for the following reasons. The best clinicians and strongest researchers are providing clinical services and conducting research. Furthermore, staff training and awareness about new procedures and technology followed by improved client care are direct results. Both lead to the establishment of a rewarding, stimulating professional environment which contributes to improved staff recruitment and retention.

There is also an ethical reason for accepting the challenge of doing research. The speech-language pathologist is frequently asked by clients or their relatives, "Does this treatment actually work?" This question is very difficult to answer ethically and truthfully without controlled research to substantiate an affirmative response. Ferketic (1993) stated, "We can't ignore the challenge to promote efficacy research. There are many questions to be answered. We all have something to offer and we need to work together to answer the questions. It's an opportunity to strengthen our professional credibility and viability" (p. 12). Collaboration between researchers and clinicians has been identified as a priority by the American Speech and Hearing Foundation (ASHF) and the National Institute on Deafness and Other Communication Disorders (Ferketic, 1993). Siegel (1993) calls research on efficacy "a natural bridge between the requirements of careful research and the needs of clinical practice" (p. 37). It is the premise of this book that the clinician should be engaged in research and the researcher should be sensitive to the need for researching questions related to clinical efficacy. Dr. John J. O'Neill, past president of the American Speech-Language-Hearing Association (ASHA), projected the need for communication between researchers and clinicians when he required all speech-language pathology and audiology graduate students at the University of Illinois to meet weekly so that those conducting research could present their projects and the clinicians and other researchers in attendance could question every aspect of the studies including their potential for contribution to clinical practice (personal communication, 1968–1969). This practice should be a part of every university program and undergraduate students should be included in the exercise. Students also need instruction in reading and evaluating journal articles.

Research Training: Setting the Stage for Lifelong Learning

It invariably amuses an experienced professor to overhear an undergraduate student comment that "after graduation I am never going to read or write another thing!" The speech-language pathologist who is truly committed to providing quality services to clients and to continuing education likely reads and writes more following graduation than while in training. Lifelong continuing education is an important component of professional responsibility. As Moll (1983) so effectively stated, "graduate education should be viewed as only an interim stage of a total continuum of education" (p. 26). The major stages of research training and experience are included in Figure 1–1. Furthermore, the ASHA Code of Ethics (ASHA, 1993a) invokes the holders of the Certificate of Clinical Competence to "continue their professional development throughout their careers" (p. 17). What better way to continue one's professional development than through the activities involved in research?

Bardach and Kelly (1991) described most research as being "the continuation if not the repetition of previously performed studies" (p. 132). Thus, reviewing the literature and previous studies about a topic prior to conducting an additional project is an excellent continuing education exercise.

Each time a student or clinician reviews the literature about a particular communication disorder in an effort to develop an appropriate treatment program for a client, a form of research is under way. Furthermore, a review of the literature often sparks interest in a topic that needs further investigation. The reviewer ultimately must become an astute consumer of published research (Pannbacker, Lass, & Middleton, 1988). This, too, is a continuing education process because published articles vary widely in scope, depth, quality, and validity (Rosenfeld, 1991).

What to Look for in a Research Training Program

Siegel (1993) expressed concern that the number of master's degree programs in speech-language pathology requiring students to complete original research is shrinking. This may be an artifact of increased enrollment accompanied incongruously by the more limited resources experienced by universities throughout the nation during the 1990s. Regardless of whether an original research project is required in a student's program, every student should graduate with the knowledge and skills needed to conduct research. Furthermore, students should view research as a process that can be integrated into daily clinical activity rather than as the tedious task of completing an expansive product.

The student who is serious about learning to do research may find many opportunities within the training program. The student might first review the research productivity of the program's faculty. One way to

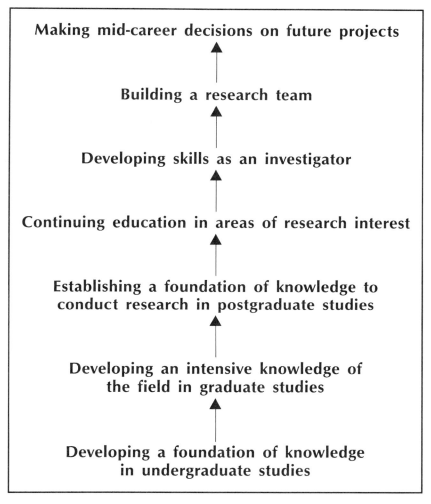

Making mid-career decisions on future projects

▲

Building a research team

▲

Developing skills as an investigator

▲

Continuing education in areas of research interest

▲

Establishing a foundation of knowledge to
conduct research in postgraduate studies

▲

Developing an intensive knowledge of
the field in graduate studies

▲

Developing a foundation of knowledge
in undergraduate studies

FIGURE 1–1. Major stages in research training and experience. (From "The research career ladder in human communication sciences and disorders" by C. L. Ludlow, 1986. In R. McLaughlin [Ed.], *Speech-language pathology and audiology: Issues and management* [pp. 409–424]. New York: Grune & Statton, with permission).

do this is to do a computer search at the library of faculty members' publications. Once a student identifies the faculty who are doing research and the specific topics they are researching, the student might consider asking to enroll in a project or independent study class under the direction of a particular professor who is actively conducting research of interest to the student. Students often develop basic skills in research by assisting with faculty research projects. Students who are required or elect to complete a thesis project should begin the project early. A thesis director from the faculty should be identified and groundwork begun on a project during the first year of the student's graduate program.

Library holdings should support research projects of interest to the student. If library holdings are incomplete, the student may need to collect information by interlibrary loan. Such requests must be made early so that projects can be completed on time. Students also need to identify available computer support for processing statistical data and word processing. Most universities have computer laboratories in libraries and instructional learning centers. Some even have computers for student use in the dormitories.

If a student is interested in doing a project that requires extraordinary expense, the location of research funding should be investigated. Many universities have projects and grants offices that may be of assistance. The department in which the student is enrolled also may have research funds available.

A research methods course in speech-language pathology is an essential element in the curriculum of a program accredited in speech-language pathology by the Educational Standards Board (ESB) of the American Speech-Language-Hearing Association (ASHA, 1992a). The student who enrolls in the research course while an undergraduate or early in the master's program has an advantage in the development of research skills. The course should be taught by a faculty member who is an active researcher and who is committed to mentoring students. Individual conferences with students about their projects are an essential part of this course. Students should make their appointments early and be prepared with ideas and strategies for conducting a project.

Practicing professionals with limited research skills should not view this condition as permanent. Research training is available through seminars, postgraduate fellowships, and involvement with a mentor who is an active and experienced researcher. Findley and DeLisa (1990) provide the types of instruction that should be included in the curriculum for research training programs and advice to individuals about selecting such training programs.

How to Continue Doing Research
After Completing Training

After completion of training, graduates generally view professional employment and beginning the Clinical Fellowship Year (CFY) as top priorities. When selecting a supervisor for the CFY, graduates might determine the research interests and activities of available supervisors. Furthermore, individuals with similar questions and research interests should be identified.

Establishment of a research team is an efficient means of beginning to conduct research. When members of a research team bring to the process an array of skills and interests, the process becomes less time consuming and tedious for individual members.

Once a team of researchers becomes efficient and productive, they need to consider their obligation to the mentoring of others. Willingness of a team to include new members is an important aspect of professional responsibility for the future. A fringe benefit of working on a research team is the establishment of lifelong friendships.

Findley and DeLisa (1990) recommend that beginning researchers select research questions that correspond closely to their regular clinical practice. This provides an opportunity to "balance empathy and clinical intuition with objectivity and observation" (p. 327). Furthermore, with the presence of colleagues interested in the results of the studies conducted on the site, the researcher tends to finish projects more quickly. If research is understood to be part of one's clinical activity, there is no need to feel guilty about time spent on research rather than provision of clinical services or vice versa. Both are considered equally important.

HISTORICAL EVOLUTION OF RESEARCH IN COMMUNICATION DISORDERS

During the academic year 1968–1969, the author was a teaching assistant for Dr. Elaine Pagel Paden at the University of Illinois. During that year, Paden supervised her teaching staff in Illinois from Washington DC where she spent weeks in the basement of the old American Speech-Language-Hearing Association (ASHA) headquarters at 9030 Old Georgetown Road sorting through dusty boxes of historical documents. Her charge by ASHA's Executive Council was to write a history of the then-named American Speech and Hearing Association. She and her committee diligently put together an interesting and entertaining historical summary that covers the years 1925–1958. Included in the book are photographs of the founders of the association. These are of special interest and sentimental value to long-term ASHA members. Following is a summary of the early efforts by the membership to compile completed projects and continue research in speech disorders as described in Paden's (1970) history.

A small group interested in speech disorders met, beginning in 1919, at the annual meeting of the National Association of Teachers of Speech (NATS) until 1925. Lee Edward Travis reported a study in which he described the effects on phonatory pitch of stutterers and nonstutterers following the firing of a blank pistol at close range without warning. The teachers of public address (public speaking) in attendance were outraged at such inhumane treatment of subjects under investigation. Following this incident it was decided that a separate organization for individuals interested in researching speech disorders should be established.

In December of 1925 the American Academy of Speech Correction was organized by 11 individuals, 5 men and 6 women. Conducting research about speech disorders was one of the three minimal requirements for membership. From the very beginning, the group emphasized the importance of a working, productive organization. The projects initially assigned to the membership were all research in nature. They included establishing the classifications and terminology for the field, summarizing thesis projects in progress, developing bibliographies on topics in speech correction, and investigating topics including stuttering, foreign accent problems, and phonetic description of "careless speech".

Realizing the need for a vehicle for publishing studies in speech correction, the group initially mimeographed 28 studies and made them available for $3.00 each. Having made money on the project, the group continued the practice. The *Journal of Speech Disorders* was established in 1935. The University of Illinois library has in its collection the early issues of this journal. While a student there, the author enjoyed many hours reading the early studies and reports.

In the first issue of the new journal published in 1936, three articles appeared covering the topics foreign dialect, cleft palate, and stuttering. Also a bibliography covering speech, voice, and hearing disorders was included. Gradually the journal became less devoted to news items and increasingly dedicated to quality scholarly content. The camaraderie and friendships established among the young and energetic contributors with similar professional interests remained.

Eventually the *Journal of Speech Disorders* was renamed *Journal of Speech and Hearing Disorders*. The majority of articles that appeared in the journal for the first 20 years covered topics on stuttering followed by articles on general topics and therapy and "audiometry." Also, between 1936 and 1949, the articles were more clinically oriented. In 1950, the journal's focus shifted to articles with a research orientation until 1957 when the reverse trend began.

With the explosion of submitted research, the *Journal of Speech and Hearing Research* (JSHR) began publication in 1958. This journal adopted a research orientation while the *Journal of Speech and Hearing Disorders* (JSHD) published research with clinical application. Because individuals working in school settings were interested in clinical applications and felt that neither journal served their needs, another ASHA journal, *Language, Speech, Hearing Services in Schools* (LSHSS), began publication in 1970.

In an effort to increase the relevance of the ASHA journal program to all members, in 1990 the *Journal of Speech and Hearing Disorders* was combined with the *Journal of Speech and Hearing Research* and its title was discontinued. Two new journals were initiated. The *American Journal of Audiology: A Journal of Clinical Practice* and the *American Journal of Speech-language Pathology: A Journal of Clinical Practice* were first published in the fall of 1991. With these changes, both audiologists and speech-language pathologists have subject specific periodicals in which to publish clinical and experimental research. One of the first projects students majoring in speech-language pathology should undertake is to become familiar with the professional journals provided by ASHA to its membership.

FUTURE DIRECTIONS OF RESEARCH IN COMMUNICATION DISORDERS

As accountability for therapy outcome continues to be required by insurance companies, families, and clients, it is paramount that controlled, reliable treatment research be given a high priority by speech-language pathologists and audiologists. Clinicians cannot afford to assume that "others will do it" because others may not choose to research questions relevant to specific clinical practice needs.

Based on the recent changes in ASHA journals and the increased demand for efficacy-based research, more clinical research conducted by clinicians in the professional setting appears imminent. Furthermore, during the past decade, a rising number of female speech-language pathologists have published projects in ASHA journals. Middleton and Pannbacker (unpublished) studied research productivity in ASHA journals according to author gender from 1960 to 1991. They found that research productivity in ASHA publications has not reflected gender representation of ASHA membership. The percent of female authors publishing in *JSHR*, *JSHD*, and *Asha* ranged from 32.4% to 38.7%. However, female authors comprised 57.9% of those publishing in the

LSHSS between 1970 and 1991. From 1982 to 1991, the percentage of female authors publishing in *JSHR, JSHD,* and *Asha* ranged from 43% to 49%. Female authors comprised 62.3% of those publishing in *LSHSS* between 1982 and 1991. Thus, it appears that the percentage of research projects having female authors will continue to rise.

SUMMARY

The vitality and endurance of a profession depend on the quality and quantity of its ongoing research programs. Furthermore, there are professional, ethical, and personal reasons for conducting research. Thus, it is important that students develop research skills and become astute consumers of published research. These skills are developed during academic training and should continue after graduation with the assistance of a mentor and/or a research team.

Since the profession was organized in 1925, publication of research has been actively encouraged. Publication of quality, respected professional journals has been a primary ASHA activity. The current need for research to determine efficacy of treatment creates opportunities for clinicians to become more actively involved in conducting and publishing research.

STUDY EXERCISES

1. Buy a research folder for filing completed exercises at the end of each chapter. The folder should be selected carefully. It should convey your interests, passions, or favorite leisure time activities. The author would select a folder with Garfield the cat on it, someone skiing the high country, or a scene depicting the underwater splendor observed while scuba diving. You are going to enjoy completing the exercises in this book. Your research folder should convey a positive personal message.

2. Type and sign the following contract using your word processor. This should comprise the first page in your research folder.

   I, (print your full name), the undersigned do seriously and in sound mind agree that I possess the curiosity, the professional commitment and dedication, and the ability to learn the methodology for doing research and to become skilled in the technical aspects of completing research projects. I further understand that the recognition and intrinsic and extrinsic rewards for doing research are *not* reserved for graduate faculty members with many years of experience. If I begin my research career early, I may make some important contributions to the profession. While conducting my research, I will enjoy learning, discovering, developing important friendships with colleagues, and providing information that will help not just my clients but all clients served by speech-language pathologists familiar with my research. I enthusiastically begin my research career.

_____   _____

Signature   Date

3. Locate the journals published by the American Speech-Language-Hearing Association in your university library. In what year do they begin? Compare the older journals in format and content with the most current ones. Be efficient in time management by completing the next exercise while doing this one.

4. List at least three topics you are interested in researching.

   Example: The results of operant versus combined management programming for adult stutterers.

   Provide a list of references that you consulted to select your topics. Use a word processor to do this assignment. Make sure the reference list is completed in the same format as those listed at the end of articles in current ASHA journals.

5. Show your list of topics to another student or to a colleague. What were the responses of that person toward your selections? Were you given any additional ideas? What were they? File your list in your folder.

6. Make an appointment with a faculty member in your program for the purpose of discussing research projects being conducted by faculty. Prepare a list of questions you plan to ask prior to going to the interview. File your questions and an outline of the answers provided in your folder.

7. Read an article, book, or monograph written by a faculty member in your program. Look at the names of the co-authors and individuals mentioned in the acknowledgments section. Does it appear that students may have assisted with the project?

8. Locate computer support on your campus. File in your folder the location, telephone number, and the name of a person on site who will be willing to assist you.

SUGGESTED READINGS

American Speech-Language-Hearing Association. (1993). Code of ethics. *Asha*, *35*(3), 17–18.

Ferketic, M. (1993). Professional practices perspective on efficacy. *Asha*, *35*(1), 12.

Siegel, G. (1993). Research: A natural bridge. *Asha*, *35*(1), 36–37.

CHAPTER 2

ETHICS AND SCIENTIFIC RESEARCH

MARY H. PANNBACKER AND DAVID L. IRWIN

- The Need for Ethical Guidelines
- Ethical Issues
- Institutional Review Boards
- Summary
- Study Exercises
- Suggested Readings

In recent years, ethical issues of research have received greater attention because of unethical practices and greater awareness of fraud and scientific inaccuracy (ASHA, 1991c; Drew & Hardman, 1985; Frohlich, 1993; Holzemer, 1988; Resnick, 1993; Schiedermayer & Siegler, 1986). Most disciplines have established codes of ethics which include standards of ethical conduct in research. The Code of Ethics of the American Speech-Language-Hearing Association (1993a) contains four specific references to ethics in research:

> Individuals shall use persons in research or as subjects of teaching demonstrations only with their informed consent. (p. 17)

> Individuals' statements to the public—advertising, announcing, and marketing their professional services, reporting research results, and promoting products—shall adhere to prevailing professional standards and shall not contain misrepresentations. (p. 18)

> Individuals' statements to colleagues about professional services, research results, and products shall adhere to prevailing professional standards and shall contain no misrepresentations. (p. 18)

> Individuals shall assign credit only to those who have contributed to a publication, presentation, or product. Credit shall be assigned in proportion to the contribution and only with the contributor's consent. (p. 18)

In other words, it is considered unethical to: (1) use individuals in research or in teaching demonstrations without their informed consent; (2) make statements to the public or colleagues, including reporting the results of research that does not adhere to prevailing professional standards or contains misrepresentations; (3) inappropriately assign credit(s) for publication(s) or presentation(s); and (4) assign credit without the contributor's consent.

Consideration of ethical issues related to research is extremely important for both the beginning and experienced researcher as well as the consumer of research. The purpose of this chapter is to consider these issues and the role of Institutional Review Boards in protecting research subjects.

THE NEED FOR ETHICAL GUIDELINES

There has been considerable interest in the protection of human subjects since the experiments conducted with Nazi prisoners during World War II (Bordens & Abbott, 1988; Drew & Hardman, 1985). Recent cases of fraud in research continue the need for setting and enforcing ethical standards of research (Danforth & Schoenhoff, 1992; Lo, Feigal, Cummings, & Hulley, 1988). However, ethical issues in research have not always been given adequate consideration (Polit & Hungler, 1991).

ETHICAL ISSUES

The ethical issues of research involve not only the use of human subjects but the ethics of researchers, editors, consumers of research, authorship, and publication.

Subjects

The rights of human subjects are a major ethical consideration in research (Braddom, 1990). Research on human subjects is justified only if the benefits to be derived outweigh the risks taken (Garrett, Bailie, & Gorga, 1989). Other issues include not exposing subjects to physical or psychological harm, not deceiving subjects about the purpose of the research, and not divulging private confidential information about the subjects (Doehring, 1988). For further information about these issues, the interested reader is referred to Bordens and Abbott (1988), Drew and Hardman (1985), Kidder and Judd (1986), Lo et al. (1988), Metz and Folkins (1985), Polit and Hungler (1991), and Sieber (1993). Similar ethical considerations apply to the use of animals in research (Folkins, Gorga, Luschei, Vetter, & Watson, 1993).

Researchers, Editors, and Consumers of Research

Research is a system that is based on trust that researchers will do scrupulous research and report it honestly, that editorial reviewers will objectively review manuscripts, and that editors will treat authors without favoritism or bias (Caelleigh, 1991). The ethics of the consumer will also be discussed.

Researchers

The responsibilities of researchers include high ethical standards in designing and conducting research, intellectual honesty, integrity, and responsible co-authorship (Huth, 1990; Leedy, 1989; Schiedermayer &

Siegler, 1986; Sigma Xi, 1991). The researcher's first ethical responsibility is to design research which provides usable information to answer questions. Furthermore, honesty is as important in research as it is in clinical practice. The elements of intellectual honesty involve reporting only what researchers mean and providing negative and counter evidence as well as evidence that favors their viewpoint(s). Researchers are obligated to credit others accurately for their work. All work is built on the contributions of others; these contributions should be acknowledged (Luey, 1987).

Editors

According to Caelleigh (1993) "editors have important but indirect roles in sustaining integrity in research, and they have major and highly visible roles in maintaining the integrity" of scientific literature (p. 523). The first responsibility of the editor is to the readers (Goldwyn, 1990). Other responsibilities of editors and editorial reviewers include selecting meaningful contributors to the literature and treating authors ethically relative to confidentiality, impartiality, and courtesy. Editors are also responsible for protecting authors from indiscriminate or unduly harsh reviewers, and protecting reviewers from aggravated authors (Caelleigh, 1991). Violations of confidentiality, impartiality, and courtesy by editors or reviewers undermine the credibility of scholarly publications (Schiedermayer & Siegler, 1986).

Editors and reviewers should maintain confidentiality in dealing with authors; a submitted manuscript is a privileged communication. Confidentiality protects the "author's intellectual property" (Schiedermayer & Siegler, 1986, p. 2044).

Editorial review should be a method of assessing and improving a manuscript; it should not be discriminatory or inhibitory. Appropriate editorial reviews represent the views of qualified experts who use editorial guidelines to determine the merits of an author's manuscript and its potential use (Kornblut, 1988). Editorial review "can save an author from mistakes of fact, poor logic, ignorance of sources, and other embarrassments" (Luey, 1987, p. 14). According to the American Speech-Language-Hearing Association (ASHA, 1990c) editorial review "maximizes the likelihood that serious error of fact, reasoning, or method will be detected and eliminated" (p. 4). In other words, editorial review is a method for assessing and improving a manuscript, particularly as it relates to the journal for which it has been submitted (Kornblut, 1988).

Avoiding bias in the editorial review is an important issue. The author and reviewer may be rivals, and even anonymous reviewers may find it difficult to review a paper that conflicts with their own views. Impartiality facilitates publication of a broad range of papers and makes journals worth reading.

Consumers of Research

All speech-language pathologists and audiologists should be consumers of research (Silverman, 1993). The ability of speech-language pathologists and audiologists to critically read the literature is a necessary and fundamental skill for both clinicians and researchers. Reading is an important method of continuing education and a method of learning about important advances in speech-language pathology and audiology and improvements in treatment of communication disorders. The ability to read critically allows speech-language pathologists and audiologists to analyze data and make informed decisions about what to accept and what to reject. Hegde (1994) warns that uncritical reading of the literature "is likely to perpetuate the use of less effective or ineffective assessment and treatment procedures" as well as making "permanent victims of faddish change in theory and practice" (p. 412). Furthermore, critically reading the literature allows speech-language pathologists and audiologists to read selectively and more efficiently, making more effective use of discretionary time (Alguire, Massa, Leinhart, & Henry, 1988).

Consumers of research should read the literature critically because all publications are not equal; there is considerable variation in the quality of published research. Publication is no guarantee of quality; both good and inadequate or marginal papers are published (Bardach & Kelly, 1991; Bordens & Abbott, 1988; Gates, 1991; Ventry & Schiavetti, 1986). Most of the published literature has weaknesses and limitations (Polit & Hungler, 1991). Unfortunately, some readers have the impression that a paper that is published must be reliable; these readers may become victims of bad products and faddish claims. Readers can improve their clinical practice by becoming better consumers of research (Findley, 1989; Garrett et al., 1989). Kuzma (1984) points out that "it is a well-known, but regrettable, fact that some research literature is of poor quality. After wading through a mire of jargon, inconsistencies, poor grammar, tangles of qualifications, and some muddy logic, the user is expected to draw a brilliantly clear scientific conclusion. This problem is chronic in much scientific writing"

(p. 224). Venolia (1987) feels that "slipshod writing breeds distrust," and prompts "readers to wonder if language is the writer's only area of incompetence" (p. 2). Ventry and Schiavetti (1986) believe "the appearance of an article in a journal is no guarantee of the article's quality. There is good research, and there is poor research, both of which may be published" (p. 18). Readers should respond by writing letters to the editors of journals praising, condemning, or otherwise commenting on articles (Lundberg & Williams, 1991; Silverman, 1993).

Critically reviewing the published literature is a skill that requires background knowledge and is acquired through training and experience (Doehring, 1988). Coury (1991) suggested a simple strategy for critically reviewing journal articles which consisted of the following questions: (1) Is the article relevant? (2) Is the study methodologically sound? and (3) Do the authors reach appropriate conclusions? Review of an article should also include an examination of references (Foreman & Kirchoff, 1987). There are a number of additional ways publications can be evaluated (ASHA, 1984; Braddom, 1990; Cash, 1989; Cobb & Hagemaster, 1987; Dutwin & Diamond, 1991; Fitch, 1986; Krathwohl, 1985; Krogh, 1985; Kuzma, 1984; Riegelman, 1981; Teitelbaum, 1989). Norman (1986) believes the most important factors are scientific relevance, clarity, soundness of the experimental method, and the author(s). Both the American Psychological Association (APA) (1988) and the American Medical Association (Lundberg & Williams, 1991) have developed strategies for evaluating content. (see Table 2–1).

One prerequisite for a good researcher is the ability to critically review the literature. Furthermore, it is important to remember that reading professional journals is the most cost-efficient form of continuing education available (Gallagher, 1990).

Editorial Ethics

Ethical issues related to writing and publishing warrant discussion and analysis to ensure responsible editorial practices. There has been increased interest in these issues in recent years (Danforth & Schoenhoff, 1992; Feinstein, 1985; Schiedermayer & Siegler, 1986). In 1992, ASHA's (1992b) Ethical Practice Board stated "plagiarism, falsification, misrepresentation, fabrication, and other forms of dishonesty in scientific inquiry and scientific reporting must be avoided assiduously, and any and all instances of fraud and fakery in research and scholarship will be considered violations of the Code of Ethics" (p. 12). Limited information about the ethics of writing and publishing is available in textbooks on research in speech-language pathology and audiology

TABLE 2–1.   Guidelines for Evaluating Quality of Content

Is the work original and important?

Does the design adequately test the hypothesis?

Are the data valid and reliable?

Are the conclusions reasonable and justified by the data?

Are subjects representative of the population to which generalizations are made?

Were ethical standards maintained?

Are the findings of interest?

Is the research developed sufficiently to make presentation of results meaningful?

Is the writing clear or can it be made clear?

Sources: Adapted from *Publication Manual of the American Psychological Association,* 1988. Washington, DC: American Psychological Association, p. 19, 20; and "The quality of a medical article" by G. D. Lundberg and E. Williams, 1991, *Journal of the American Medical Association, 265,* 1161–1162.

(Doehring, 1988; Hegde, 1994; Shearer, 1982; Silverman, 1993; Ventry & Schiavetti, 1986). Speech-language pathologists and audiologists need to be knowledgeable about these issues if they are to be responsible authors, editors, and consumers of research. The purpose of this section is to review issues related to editorial ethics including "publish or perish," fraud and deception, irresponsible authorship, redundant publication, plagiarism, editorial prejudice, and publication bias which are illustrated in Figure 2–1.

Publish or Perish

Publication is essential to academic survival, that is, promotion, tenure, and merit pay in academia. Thus, speech-language pathologists and audiologists in colleges and universities may feel impelled to publish as frequently as possible (Anderson, 1992; Boyes, Happel, & Hogan, 1984; Diamond, 1989; Morgan, 1984; Schaefer, 1990). Pressures to publish can lead to deceptive practices such as reporting the same study in installments (least publishable unit), more than once (self-plagiarism), and listing people as authors who were only marginally involved in the study (honorary authors). Angell (1986) believes these problems could be reduced by limiting the number of publications considered in evaluation for promotion or funding. Some universities have guidelines for

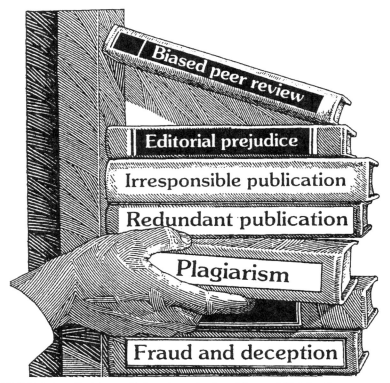

FIGURE 2-1. Problems Related to Authorship and Publication.

the maximum number of publications considered for appointment or promotion to each faculty level: five for assistant professor, seven for associate professor, and ten for full professor (Committee on Responsible Conduct of Research, 1989). This practice encourages emphasis on quality not quantity of publications, in other words, fewer publications but ones that make significant contributions to the body of knowledge.

Fraud and Deception

Fraud is a major ethical abuse which, according to Braxton (1991), violates three or more of the four norms of science: universalism, communality, disinterestedness, and organized skepticism. These norms are described in Table 2–2. Fraud is sophisticated dishonesty which is difficult to detect but, if detected, usually catches the attention of

TABLE 2–2. The Four Norms of Science and Violations Classified According to the Norm Violated

Norm	Description	Violations
Universalism	Findings of research must not be assessed on the basis of particularistic criteria such as race, nationality, class, or personal qualities. Also, scientific careers should be predicated on merit or talent rather than on particularistic criteria.	1. Accorded high standing to a scholar, not on the basis of scientific merit, but because of personal or social characteristics (race, gender, prestige of institutional affiliation). 2. Used scholar's past work as a basis for assessing that person's current scholarship. 3. Rejected theory or research findings because of the author's social or personal characteristics. 4. Circulated preprints or reprints of research to others based on social or personal characteristics of such individuals.
Communality	Findings of research must be made public because such findings are the property of the research community. Specifically, secrecy about ongoing research is prohibited; recognition of the contribution of a scholar by others is preferred.	1. Kept research findings secret. 2. Failed to inform others investigating similar topics about their current work. 3. Failed to give proper citation or reference to pertinent published work of others. 4. Failed to give credit to the contribution of a collaborator.

(continued)

TABLE 2–2. *(continued)*

Norm	Description	Violations
Disinterestedness	Prohibits the individual from doing research for the primary purpose of receiving recognition from colleagues or gaining prestige and financial reward from the lay community. The preferred motive for research is advancing knowledge.	1. Engaged in a scholarly or research project for the sole purpose of financial gain or personal recognition. 2. Knowingly published research containing errors. 3. Knowingly published research with fraudulent data or materials. 4. Named a law, effect, or procedure after themselves. 5. Sought publicity for research findings from the mass media.
Organized Skepticism	No knowledge claim or research finding should be accepted without assessment based on empirical and logical criteria (i.e., individual professionals should take a critical view toward scholarly contributions and research findings).	1. Ignored critical peer review of scholarship and research. 2. Used research or scholarly work of others without critical review. 3. Remained committed to own research findings despite evidence contradicting such findings. 4. Rejected theory or research finding because it differed from current disciplinary thought. 5. Failed to present data contradicting own research findings. 6. Accepted own research findings as valid prior to critical peer review. 7. Failed to question own research findings when others were unable to replicate findings. 8. Made a personal attack on the work of a colleague which is in conflict with their own work.

Source: Adapted from "The influence of graduate department quality on the sanctions of scientific misconduct" by J. Braxton, 1991, *Journal of Higher Education, 62,* 87–108.

the public press. Friedman (1990) believes it is difficult to correct fraudulent publication because journals rarely have policies and procedures for responding to allegations of improper research. Pfeifer and Snodgrass (1990) described several reasons why invalid information is used including "a dearth of available information on retracted works: inconsistency in retraction format, terminology, and indexing and an apparent lack of sufficient attention to manuscripts by some authors and editors" (p. 1420). On the other hand, Garfield and Welliams-Dorof (1990) feel the "literature seems to purge itself of articles that are known or even suspected to be fraudulent" (p. 1426). It is now easier to identify improprieties in the published literature because when an author or editor retracts a previous publication by means of a formally printed notification such notices are indexed in the National Library of Medline's MEDLINE data base as RETRACTION OF PUBLICATION, while the original article, to which the retraction refers, is indexed RETRACTED PUBLICATION (Duggar, 1993). In 1993, the *National Institute of Health Guide for Grants and Contracts* (U.S. Department of Health and Human Services) began publication of findings of scientific misconduct. This serves both educational and deterrent purpose(s). Additional sanctions for dealing with scientific misconduct have been described by Dresser (1993), Korenman (1993), and Shore (1993).

Instances of scientific misconduct also involve fraud. Some examples include irresponsible authorship; wasteful publication; honorary authorship; failure to explain the limitations in data; selective, fragmentary, or inaccurate reporting of findings; and fabricating or plagiarizing data (Silverman, 1992).

The first step in reducing these problems is a periodic review of ethical standards. Other steps include more restraint in the use of questionable practices, full disclosure and justification for using questionable practices, and "greater skepticism by readers" (Bailar, 1986, p. 259). Skepticism by co-authors and editors may also be effective in reducing and eliminating questionable practices.

Irresponsible Authorship

There are several problems related to authorship that warrant consideration including unjustified authorship, incomplete authorship, and errors relative to quotations or references. Unjustified authors are individuals who made suggestions, but did not take part in the research, help write the manuscript, or review the final draft submitted for publication. In other words, unjustified authors do not contribute substantially to the work (Committee on Responsible Conduct of Research,

1989; Cowell, 1989; Davenport, 1990; Kalichman & Friedman, 1992). Some examples of unjustified or gift authorship include the department head who did not contribute to the research; the dissertation committee who reviewed the dissertation; and the first author's spouse who has a degree in library science and gathered information from clinical records.

Incomplete authorship is probably rare (Huth, 1986). This type of irresponsible authorship is failure to include individuals as authors who had responsibility for important content of a manuscript (Huth, 1986). The most usual examples are a student's dissertation advisor who fails to include the student as an author or a student who does not include an adviser who has made a substantial contribution (Madsen, 1992). The ASHA Code of Ethics (1993a) addresses the issue of authorship by stating "individuals should assign credit to those who have contributed to a publication in proportion to their contribution" (p. 18).

An individual's approval should be obtained before he or she is listed as an author (O'Connor & Woodford, 1977). Any individual who makes a major contribution to a manuscript should be listed as an author. Authorship includes not only those who do the actual writing but also those who have made other substantial contributions (American Psychological Association, 1988). Individuals who simply advised or provided technical assistance in the usual course of their work are not included as authors. One's department head or other senior colleagues should not be included as authors unless they made significant contributions to the research.

The order of authorship should be determined in relation to the degree of contribution (Drew & Hardman, 1985; Risenberg & Lundberg, 1990; Waltz, Nelson, & Chambers, 1985). The individual making the greatest contribution should be first author and the others listed in order of their relative contributions. If the contributions are relatively equal, the order of authorship can be determined alphabetically, by a flip of the coin, or some other method that is mutually agreeable. Members of research teams often take turns as senior or first author. An exception to these practices is when a journal requires alphabetical order.

There are also other issues related to irresponsible authorship. One issue is the accuracy of references and quotations. It is the author's responsibility to verify the accuracy of all references and quotations. Many authors do not verify references and quotations because errors are common in the published literature (DeLacey, Record, & Wade, 1985; Doms, 1989; Eichorn & Yankauer, 1987; Evans, Nadjari, & Burchell, 1990; Foreman & Kirchoff, 1987). Henson (1990) knows of an editor who will not "send a manuscript out for review if it violates any referencing rules" (p. 801). DeLacey, Record, and Wade (1985) believe editors should sample references for accuracy; if any error is found, the manuscript should be returned to the author(s) with instructions to verify the accuracy of all references. The *Pharos,* the journal published by the AOA honorary medical society, requires authors to provide copies of all articles cited or referenced in manuscripts (Hoekelman, 1992).

Redundant Publication

The extreme of redundant publication is self-plagiarism, which is publication of essentially the same article in different professional journals (Angell & Relman, 1989; Brier & Fulginiti, 1990). Sometimes known as double or triple publishing this practice is "considered to be a cardinal sin against the ethics of science" (Day, 1988, p. 147). It is an outrage to readers, a nuisance to editors, and a threat to publishers who are legally responsible for copyright violations (Goldwyn, 1990). It also wastes space and the resources of the peer-review system as well as distorting the reward system. Redundant publication is a way of gaining unearned credit for productivity; thus it is misleading (Angell & Relman, 1989). Editors should: (1) require authors to verify that a manuscript has not been accepted or published elsewhere and (2) ask reviewers to cite prior publication of the content of the manuscript under review (Huth, 1986).

Related to redundant publication is duplicate or multiple submission of a manuscript, in other words, simultaneously submitting a manuscript for publication to more than one journal. Many journals require authors to affirm that the manuscript is not under consideration in another journal (ASHA, 1990c).

Fragmented Publication

Fragmented publication is the division of a single research project into a string of papers each of which is referred to as the "least publishable unit" (Angell, 1986; Huth, 1986). Goldwyn (1990) refers to this type of author as a "salami slicer" who has his or her name on several papers when one would have been enough (p. 281). Huth (1986) believes divided publication is difficult to deal with and that editors cannot do much about it.

Plagiarism

Taking someone else's work and presenting it as one's own can be deliberate or unintentional. Plagiarism, even when it is unintentional, is inexcusable (Madsen, 1992). Klein (1993) suggests "that plagiarism is scientific misconduct because the rewards of science are so heavily dependent on evidence of primacy and originality" (p. 57). Plagiarism can be word-for-word (exact) or patchwork, that is, a single word is changed but the information otherwise is quoted verbatim without citing the reference as a direct quotation. Plagiarism can be avoided by making certain that complete, accurate citations are given for direct and indirect quotations, statistical data, graphs, tables, and so on. Authors should be familiar with the appropriate procedure for citing references as presented in the *Publication Manual of the American Psychological Association* (American Psychological Association, 1988), *The Simon and Schuster Handbook for Writers* (Troyka, 1990), or the *Chicago Manual of Style* (University of Chicago, 1982). Using another person's work without giving credit may go beyond plagiarism into copyright infringement (Luey, 1987).

Closely related to plagiarism is lazy writing. In lazy writing, the author takes multiple paragraphs from one or more sources and presents them as a paper. Lazy writing differs from plagiarism in that the author properly cites the references (Bordens & Abbott, 1988; Weidenborner & Caruso, 1982). This practice is not compatible with scholarship (Woodford, 1989a).

Publication Bias

Publication of a manuscript is the result of a long, complex process. Many people, acting as investigators, members of institutional review boards, authors, reviewers, and editors make decisions that influence what is published. According to Rennie and Flanagin (1992), "each decision may be subject to biases; the conscious and subconscious influences that interfere with impartial judgments" (p. 411).

Blank and McElmurry (1988) believe publication review practices are of questionable objectivity because

> Editors hold almost total control over what is and is not published; most do the initial screening of manuscripts, rejecting out of hand those that do not fit publication criteria; they choose the review panel, and the particular individuals who are asked to critique each manuscript; and the ultimate decision to

publish or not to publish an article rests in their hands; the possibility for personal bias or mutual socialization in editorial decision making is apparent. (p. 181)

Ventry and Schiavetti (1986) indicated that

Not all editorial consultants have the same level of expertise, not all have comparable research or evaluation skills, not all are equally familiar with a given area, not all use the same standards in evaluating a manuscript, and not all give the same amount of time and energy to the evaluation process. (pp. 17–18)

Boice and Jones (1984) reported that some academicians do not write because of discriminatory reviewing practices such as reviewers having high tolerance of papers confirming their own beliefs and the status of an author's affiliation. Several others have also described questionable publication review practices (Burham, 1990; Caelleigh, 1991; Cantekin, McGuire, & Potter, 1990; Chalmers, Frank, & Reitman, 1990; Cole, Cole, & Simon, 1981; Dickersin, 1990; Dickersin, Min, & Meinert, 1992; Sharp, 1990). The decision not to publish due to the concern that one's research will not be reviewed objectively is unfortunate.

Publication biases are less evident today than in the past (Polit & Hungler, 1991). ASHA's (1990c) reviewers are chosen to avoid conflict of interest, although they are usually chosen because they have completed previous work on specific topics. Furthermore, Dickersin, Min, and Meinert (1992) found that contrary to popular belief "publication bias originates primarily with investigators, not journal editors" (p. 374). O'Connor and Woodford (1977) believe most reviewers are impartial in their evaluation of manuscripts and "too busy to spend time and effort inventing trivial objections" (p. 71). Editorial reviewers should be competent in the field they review, which includes being familiar with current research, able to objectively review other people's work, willing to spend the time necessary to review manuscripts, make useful comments, and do all of this within a deadline (Luey, 1987).

Rennie (1990) states that the peer review process "has become one of the most important quality-control mechanisms in science" (p. 1317). Researchers are so concerned about peer review that an International Congress on Peer Review was held in 1989. A second congress was held in September, 1991 (Lundberg & Williams, 1991). Sharp (1990) provided several suggestions for reducing reviewer bias such as a "blind" peer review, an "open" review by removing anonymity, sending out every paper for review, checks on fraud, an appeal mechanism, obtaining integrity statements from reviewers, providing a structured means of review such as a questionnaire or checklist, and increasing the number of reviewers from one or two to several.

Conclusions

Speech-language pathologists and audiologists have an ethical obligation to know about responsible writing and publishing practices. Both the researcher and the consumer of research should recognize that:

1. Appropriate attention should be given to ethical issues at professional meetings and in publications.
2. There should be training in responsible research conduct.
3. All readers have the responsibility to critically review the literature.
4. Authors should appropriately manage pressures to publish.
5. Each author should be able to document his or her contribution to a paper.
6. Authors should accurately cite and quote others' works.
7. Authors should remember that editors and reviewers can save them from making mistakes.
8. Editorial review should be fair and impartial.
9. Editors and reviewers should have uniform standards for evaluating manuscripts.
10. Reviewers should be willing to spend the time necessary to review manuscripts.
11. Editors and reviewers have the responsibility to acknowledge conflicts of interest.
12. Editors should be willing to accept authorized retractions or corrections.
13. Editors have a responsibility to develop written policies and procedures for responding to allegations of research misconduct.
14. Authors and editors should avoid redundant publication.
15. Editors and reviewers have the responsibility to sample the accuracy of references and quotations.

Speech-language pathologists and audiologists should be aware of strategies for resolving ethical problems related to research. Seymour (1994) has provided general suggestions for identification and resolution of ethical problems (see Figure 2–2).

INSTITUTIONAL REVIEW BOARDS

This section is concerned with Institutional Review Boards (IRBs). The IRB is an integral part of the protection of human subjects in research

What is the problem/conflict/dilemma?
- Is it a professional violation?
- Is it a legal violation?
- Is it both a professional and legal violation?

What values are in conflict?
- Under these circumstances, what is of most value?
- Will feelings interfere with judgment?

What evidence is provided by the parties involved?
- Whose evidence is most convincing?
- Is there consistency in the evidence?
- Has all the evidence been heard?
- What is acceptable practice in this situation?
- Who is most believable?
- Have other view points been considered?

What action can be taken or recommended?
- Is outside consultation needed?
- What are the social, cultural and political impacts of the consequences?
- What are the short- and long-term impacts of the consequences?

In whose best interest is the decision?
- Will the decision be fair to all parties concerned?
- If yes, why? If no, why not?

How will the decision impact the present and the future?

FIGURE 2–2. Identification and Resolution of Ethical Dilemmas. (From "Ethical considerations" by C. M. Seymour [1994]. In R. Lubinski and C. Frattali [Eds.]. *Professional issues speech-language pathology and audiology: A textbook*, pp. 61–74 San Diego, CA: Singular Publishing Group, with permission.)

(Garrett et al., 1989; Metz & Folkins, 1985; Ogden, 1991; Shearer, 1982; Silverman, 1992). Almost all research in communication sciences and disorders involves the use of human subjects (Silverman, 1993). Any facility that receives federal funding, including federally sponsored fellowships, has an IRB which reviews research proposals involving human subjects. Furthermore, many facilities involved with research on human subjects require approval by an IRB, regardless of the funding source (Lo et al., 1988). IRB reviews are intended to ensure that research is ethical and protects the welfare and rights of the subjects.

Usually a facility has one IRB or human subjects committee. An IRB must have at least five members and usually consists of researchers, clinicians, patient advocates, lay members, and individuals knowledgeable about ethical and legal issues of research (Lo et al., 1988). IRB members should reflect a wide variety of backgrounds and interests (Metz & Folkins, 1985).

Before undertaking a study involving human subjects, the researcher should submit a research proposal to the IRB (Bordens & Abbott, 1988; Lo et al., 1988; Polit & Hungler, 1991). Thesis and dissertation proposals are routinely submitted to an IRB (Hegde, 1994). An informed consent form may be required as part of the research proposal. A sample consent form is presented in Figure 2–3. Sample consent forms also can be found in Bordens and Abbott (1988) and Polit and Hungler (1991).

Most IRB review is the same institution to institution (Findley, Daum, & Macedo, 1989). The major concerns of an IRB in reviewing research proposals are the risks and benefits to subjects, informed consent, and privacy and confidentiality (Hegde, 1994). An IRB may decide that certain types of research may be given expedited review, and that other types of research may be exempted from IRB review (Table 2–3). In an expedited review, a single IRB member does the review. The main requirements governing IRB decisions are summarized in Table 2–4. A proposal is more likely to be approved by an IRB at the first review if it is written clearly and succinctly elaborates on points that may be viewed critically, are easily misunderstood, or are sensitive (Tawney & Gast, 1984). An IRB can approve the proposal, require revisions, or reject the proposal. These decisions are usually documented on a review form, such as the one in Figure 2–4.

SUMMARY

In recent years greater attention has been paid to the ethical conduct of research because of past identified unethical practices. Ethical issues pertain to several aspects of the research process including obtaining informed consent from human subjects, accuracy in reporting

In signing this document, I am giving my consent to participate in a research study that will focus on the experiences and needs of families of children with hearing loss. This study is being conducted by Dr. Hannaha Willis, Professor of Communication Disorders. This study has been approved by the Institutional Review Board of Texas State University.

I understand that I will be interviewed at a time convenient to me. I will be asked some questions about my experiences as a parent of a child with a hearing loss, characteristics about this child, and my use of community resources. The interview will take about $1\frac{1}{2}$ to 2 hours to complete. I understand that the researcher may contact me for addi-tional information.

This interview was granted freely. I have been informed that the interview is entirely voluntary, and that even after the interview begins I can refuse to answer any specific questions or decide to terminate the interview at any point. I have been told that my answers to questions will not be given to anyone else and no reports of this study will identify me in any way. I have also been informed that my participation or nonparticipation or my refusal to answer questions will have no effect on services that I or any member of my family may receive from health or social services providers.

This study will help develop a better understanding of the experiences of families with children who have hearing loss. I, however, will receive no direct benefit.

I understand that the results of this study will be given to me if I ask for them and that Dr. Willis is the person to contact if I have any questions about the study or about my rights as a study participant. Dr. Willis can be reached through a collect call to (214) 797-2030.

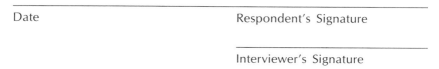

Date   Respondent's Signature

                                              Interviewer's Signature

FIGURE 2–3. Sample Consent Form. *Source:* Adapted from *Nursing Research Principles and Methods* by D. F. Polit and B. P. Hungler (1991). Philadelphia, PA: J. P. Lippincott.

research results, and properly assigning credit to investigators according to their contributions. In addition, researchers and editors should be aware of the ethics of writing and publishing. This includes maintaining confidentiality in dealing with authors, protecting intellectual property, providing objective assessment of the manuscript and suggestions for improvement, and avoiding bias in editorial review.

The consumer of research also has an ethical obligation to review research critically. Critical review involves examining references and evaluating the study for scientific relevance, clarity in presentation, soundness in methodology, and the justification for the study's conclusions based on the reported data. Fifteen specific recommendations to ensure responsible writing and publishing practices were provided to the researcher and consumer of research.

TABLE 2–3.　Exemptions From IRB Review

Surveys or interviews unless

- subjects can be identified, and
- responses could lead to legal liability, financial loss or reduced employability, and
- research deals with sensitive topics.

Observations of public behavior, except if the three conditions above apply.

Research on normal educational practices.

Studies of existing records or data, provided that the data cannot be linked to individual subjects.

Source: From "Addressing ethical issues" by B. Lo, D. Feigel, S. Cummings, and S. B. Hulley, 1988. In Hulley, S., and Cummings, S. (Eds.), *Designing clinical research* (pp. 151–158). Baltimore, MD: Williams & Wilkins, with permission. Copyright 1988 Williams & Wilkins.

TABLE 2–4.　Summary of Guidelines for IRB Decisions

Risks to subjects are minimized.

Risks to subjects are reasonable in relation to anticipated benefits, if any, to subjects and the importance of the knowledge that may reasonably be expected to result.

Selection of subjects is equitable.

Informed consent will be sought as required.

Informed consent will be appropriately documented.

Adequate provision is made for monitoring the research to ensure the safety of subject.

Appropriate provisions are made to protect the privacy of subjects and the confidentiality of data.

When vulnerable subjects are involved, appropriate safeguards are included to protect the rights and welfare of these subjects.

Source: From *Nursing Research Principles and Methods* (p. 40) by D. Polit and B. Hungler, 1991. Philadelphia: J. B. Lippincott, with permission.

A number of questionable practices were discussed in this chapter: excessive pressures on members of the academic community to

Proposal/Project Number: Internal _____ Sponsor _____

Proposal/Project Title: _____

_____

Type of Review:

_____ Determination of Exemption _____ Full Board Proposal Review

_____ Expedited Review _____ Ongoing research in certification of change

_____ Other (Please Specify): _____

After reviewing the above proposal/project:

Exemption _____ The institutional official has determined that the research is exempt under 45 CFR 46.101 (b) or

Safeguards _____ This Institutional Review Board (or member signing below in the case of expedited review) has determined by unanimous vote of the members present that:

_____ Risks to subjects are minimized and are reasonable in relation to anticipated benefits. Selection of subjects is equitable; the privacy of the subjects and confidentiality of the data are adequately protected. Approval is given.

_____ Approval is given under the following conditions:

_____ Approval is not given, for the following reasons:

Where applicable, attach summary of controversal issues and their resolution. _____

_____

Date: _____

Names of IRB Members Present   *Signatures of IRB Members Present:*

_____   _____
_____   _____
_____   _____
_____   _____
_____   _____

FIGURE 2–4. IRB Review Form. (Adapted from Nursing Research Principles and Methods by D. F. Polit and B. P. Hungler, 1991. Philadelphia: J. P. Lippincott.)

publish, fraud and deception, irresponsible authorship, redundant publication, fragmented publication, plagiarism, and publication biases. For most research, an Institutional Review Board must review the research proposal to ensure that the research is ethical and protects subjects. Thesis and dissertation proposals are routinely submitted to an IRB to determine risks and benefits of the study and the procedures for guaranteeing informed consent, privacy, and confidentiality. Guidelines governing IRB decisions were summarized.

STUDY EXERCISES

1. Obtain the form for submitting a research proposal to the Institutional Review Board (IRB) on your campus or in your hospital or clinic. Select and read a research article on a topic you selected in Exercise 4, Chapter 1. Make sure the article used humans as subjects. Pretend that you are planning to duplicate the study. Fill out the IRB proposal as completely as you can with the information available. Also, find an example of an informed consent form and include it with the assignment.

Answer the following questions as part of this exercise:

a. How does one ensure that subjects really understand the potential risk(s) when they give their consent?

b. What is the purpose of an Institutional Review Board?

c. List at least three major benefits to subjects participating in this study.

2. Read the letters to the editor about research articles in one of the journals published by ASHA. Use Tables 2–1 and 2–2 to assess content of the article that you selected for Exercise 1 above. Then, write a letter to the editor about the article in which you comment, praise, and/or condemn the study.

Include the following in your letter:

a. The major strengths (merits) and weaknesses of the study.

b. Evaluation of the extent to which you believe the researcher's discussion would facilitate utilization of the study findings clinically.

c. Suggest, if possible, clinical implications that the researchers did not discuss.

3. Review the principles of ethics in research by answering the following questions:

    a. Should the instructor of a research course teach ethical values along with research skills? Why?

    b. Are your ethics in research different from those of other aspects of your professional life? Explain.

    c. Describe the appropriate professional response if a manuscript is obviously plagiarized.

    d. How can and why should plagiarism be avoided?

    e. Differentiate between plagiarism and lazy writing. How can both be avoided?

    f. How can plagiarism be a problem even for very honest writers of research papers?

    g. Differentiate between direct and indirect quotes.

    h. Define scientific fraud and deception; explain why these concepts are important to researchers.

    i. What is the difference between fraud and scientific misconduct?

    j. What is publication bias?

    k. Compile a list of recent retractions of publications by using the Medline data base known as RETRACTION OF PUBLICATION. What subject areas do the retractions primarily involve?

4. Many professionals, particularly academicians, are expected to conduct research. Why do some resist conducting and publishing research projects?

Continue your discussion by answering the following questions:

    a. What might you do if you were about to be denied a promotion due to research inactivity?

    b. Do you feel that there should be a limit to the number of publications considered for promotion and tenure review of faculty? Explain.

c. What factors should be taken into consideration when measuring research productivity of speech-language pathologists and audiologists?

5. What is the role of the editorial staff of a journal?

Include answers to the following questions:

a. Name some of the important qualifications of a good editor; what types of activities constitute good experience for an editor?

b. Would you like to be an editor some time in your career? Why or why not?

c. How can an editor ensure fairness in editorial review and decision making?

d. How might one become more effective as an editor?

e. Explain editorial bias.

f. What kind of power does an editor exercise?

g. What is the peer review system?

h. What problems are inherent in the peer review process and how do these problems affect the published literature?

6. What errors are commonly made by consumers of research?

Include in your answer how consumers of research can improve their evaluation skills.

SUGGESTED READINGS

Beauchamp, T. L., & Childress, J. F. (1989). *Principles of biomedical ethics.* New York: Oxford University Press.

Friedman, P. J. (Ed.). (1993). Integrity in bio-medical research. *Academic Medicine, 68*(9)(Suppl.), S1–S100.

Garrett, T. M., Bailie, H. W., & Garrett, R. M. (1989). *Health care ethics.* Englewood Cliffs, NJ: Prentice-Hall.

Sigma Xi (1991). *Honor in science.* Triangle Park, NC: Sigma Xi Scientific Research Society.

CHAPTER 3

OVERVIEW OF THE RESEARCH PROCESS

GRACE F. MIDDLETON AND MARY H. PANNBACKER

- Research as a Scientific Approach
- Characteristics of Research
- Basic Research Concepts and Terms
- Collaborative Research
- The Research Process
- Common Myths About Research and How to Avoid Them
- Summary
- Study Exercises
- Suggested Readings

The research process follows established procedures so that the scientific community can readily accept findings as being valid contributions to the current pool of knowledge on the subject. However, the methodology selected for a specific project varies according to the unique aspects of a research problem (Doehring, 1988).

Beginning researchers must develop an understanding of the research process and of the specific methods available for consideration for application to a specific question. In this chapter, a discussion of the scientific approach is followed by definitions and descriptions of basic research concepts and terminology. Even when armed with basic knowledge of the terminology and methods for conducting research, many are timid about beginning projects. Collaborative research is an excellent way to begin. A discussion of the advantages and types of collaborative efforts are discussed.

Regardless of a researcher's experience and knowledge, there are certain pitfalls that most have experienced. These are often based on common myths about research. These myths and ways to avoid errors related to their acceptance are provided.

RESEARCH AS A SCIENTIFIC APPROACH

Speech-language pathology as a profession is deeply rooted in the field of psychology. It was a professor of psychology, Dean Carl E. Seashore, University of Iowa Graduate College, who instigated University of Iowa's program in speech-language pathology. He secured funding for a weekend conference, the first of its kind, to study speech disorders (Paden, 1970). In fact, the 25 charter members of the American Speech-Language-Hearing Association were primarily psychologists, physicians, and educators. As publications about speech disorders were printed in early books and journals, the members were critical of some of the work published and they became actively involved in raising professional standards by stimulating sound research based on scientific principles used in the field of psychology (Paden, 1970).

Research is conducted to answer questions and is an increasingly important component in the field of speech-language pathology and audiology because both basic and clinical questions remain unanswered. In an effort to determine cause-and-effect relationships, researchers conscientiously apply scientific methodology to carefully control variables. Because federal law governing education of handicapped children emphasizes accountability for clinical services, it is imperative that scientific methods be implemented to complete basic and applied research projects. Furthermore, the reputation of a profession depends on the quality of its research (Hegde, 1994). Experimental designs are based on the same rules for asking and answering questions regardless of the type of design selected. The rules for describing, explaining, and predicting occurrences or happenings constitute scientific method (Silverman, 1993).

Lieske (1986) described the systematic study of a problem or question as a cyclical process beginning with an unanswered question followed by a clear statement of the problem, development of appropriate hypotheses, data collection, and finally interpretation of the information gathered in an effort to reject or accept hypotheses.

Beginning with an unanswered question, the researcher first conveys the goal of the project through a clear statement of the problem. Research questions based on the problem statement must be defined in clear and precise language. Ambiguity in stating a research question leads to difficulty in answering the question. Furthermore, answers to questions and discussions involving interpretation of results must also be clearly written and defined (Silverman, 1993).

Before proceeding further, the feasibility of doing the study must be considered by determining availability of resources, time needed to complete the study, significance or applicability of the study to clinical practice or to basic knowledge underlying clinical practice, and availability of data and appropriate methodology to complete the study within ethical and legal guidelines for running human subjects or collecting confidential information (Lieske, 1986). The study then must be subjected to various tests of the application of scientific method.

A study should be capable of duplication by another researcher in an effort to confirm or deny its findings. Silverman (1993) referred to such detailed descriptions as "intersubjective testability." He described meeting the criterion for intersubjective testability as critical to the confirmation of research findings in clinical practice. Clinicians must be able to corroborate findings by duplicating the study's procedure(s) to test the claims or conclusions based on clinical studies. Inadequate confirmation of the findings of an investigation leads to serious questions about the validity or soundness of claims based on the results of the study.

When developing a study that can be interpreted as having reliable results, numbers are crucial. An adequate number of observations must be made before interpreting the results of a study as reliable. The number of observations may involve the number of subjects selected or available for the study, the number of surveys evaluated, the number of case studies analyzed, and so on. A means of calculating the reliability of information used to answer a research question should also be implemented (Silverman, 1993).

Information must be organized in a logical, coherent manner. The use of tables, graphs, charts, and figures assist in the clear and logical presentation of data. Information deemed irrelevant should not be included to reduce the chance of confusion leading to faulty or illogical conclusions. The findings generated by a study should be considered tentative or temporary based on information immediately at hand. Thus, the implications of the study's findings for future research should be stated with the idea that interpretation of the results of the current study may change with the addition of new information based on suggested subsequent studies.

In summary, research may be described as a procedure for following rules for asking and answering questions. Specifically, the rules apply to clarity in stating the research question, determining "intersubjective testability" to ascertain validity of findings, determining the reliability of findings, logically organizing relevant conclusions, and identifying implications for further research that may either confirm or reject the findings (Silverman, 1993).

CHARACTERISTICS OF RESEARCH

The reader was exposed to some of the basic characteristics of published research when research articles, monographs, and/or books were scanned and reviewed to complete the exercises at the end of Chapters 1 and 2. Following is a brief discussion of the primary factors that need to be considered when developing a research project.

The problem underlying a research project may be identified through questions raised while reading the literature; conferring with researchers, teachers, or supervisors; doing clinical work with patients; or asking questions raised by previous research (Doehring, 1988). The importance of a particular problem may not be readily evident. Sometimes major findings are accidental. However, the more evidence there is that a particular problem needs to be researched because of a gap in available knowledge, the more likely it is that the problem is important and worth researching. Careful thought and deliberation are essential to the selection of an important, relevant research problem.

The need to investigate a particular problem is justified in the written research report or article as part of the literature review, a summary of available research on a topic, and a reason for further investigation based on: (1) a void of information or (2) conflicting results in previous projects. The background information, including a literature review and the stated reason for further investigation, are summarized briefly and concisely in the final report.

Current knowledge about a topic must be considered when designing a project and interpreting its findings. Prior to selecting a project and finalizing its design, it is important to determine how much is already known or theorized about the question or problem (Doehring, 1988). After completing a research project, the findings are compared with the findings previously reported by studies of the same or similar questions.

Research in communication disorders usually tends to be directed at provisional knowledge, such as clinical applications, rather than determination of absolute truths. Thus, methods for clinical research may differ from those designed to discover universal scientific laws. However, the research question and experimental design must survive the scrutiny of peer review by individuals knowledgeable on the topic under investigation and on research methods. Ultimately, researchers must remain current on changes in research strategies to comply with and adapt to new knowledge, changing theories, new technologies accompanied by shifts in the cultural importance of spoken language in a computer age, and changes in professional practice (Doehring, 1988).

The purpose of a study is clearly stated in very specific terms and based on the design of a project and the expected answer(s) to the question(s) raised by the problem that prompted the project. The design of a study must be selected carefully to ensure that the question raised by the purpose statement can be answered by the collection of relevant data and the application of an appropriate method to treat or analyze the data. The design of a study allows the researcher to compare groups that are similar and groups that are different or to analyze specific characteristics or attributes of an individual or a group. Efficacy of treatment studies require a design to compare performance before and after specific therapy strategies have been applied. Single-subject designs are often used to study the effects of treatment or training in a clinical setting.

The procedure is the practical application of the research design. The procedure involves a description of what was done to implement the study. In a research paper or report, the procedure is described in the method section. This section should be written clearly and be so complete in its description of what was done that another researcher could duplicate the study.

A clear statement of the research problem and purpose and selection of an appropriate research design facilitates the development of a well-stated, appropriate and clear title for the project. Titles reflecting the problem, purpose, and design of a study often include specific introductory phrases. Table 3–1 provides a list of phrases often used in titles of research projects.

TABLE 3–1. Phrases Often Used in Titles of Research Projects

An Investigation of . . .
A Comparison of . . .
The Correlation Between . . .
The Relationship Between . . .
The Difference Between . . .
Differences in Perception Between . . .
The Effects of . . .
The Effectiveness of . . .
Evaluation of . . .
Assessment of . . .
An Analysis of . . .
A Study of . . .
Improving the Quality of . . .
Improving . . . Through . . .
Expectations of . . .
A Description of . . .
Trends in . . .for . . .
Factors for Consideration in . . .
Clinical Applications in . . .
The Role of the . . .
The Acquisition of . . .
The Use of . . .
The Establishment of . . .
A Content Analysis of . . .

The subjects for a study are described in the method section. All criteria used to select subjects must be specified. The method section also contains a detailed explanation of tasks the subjects performed, including descriptions of any instrumentation or tests that were utilized.

After the data have been collected, it must be analyzed. Analysis of data can be a very tedious and time-consuming process. Use of technology including the personal computer often reduces the tedium and increases the accuracy of data analysis. Once numerical data have been collected and analyzed, the results may be presented using descriptive statistics and presentation of the information on tables or in graphs. Tables and graphs should be clear and easy to interpret. If the researcher wishes to determine similarities or differences between groups or within members of one group, inferential statistics may be calculated using appropriate statistical formulae.

Some data are not converted into numerical form. Such data require qualitative analysis. Data for qualitative analysis may include narratives describing observations of behavior or information taken from discussions or exchanges. Observations involving pragmatic factors in communication are an example of such data. The method for analyzing data is reported in the method section of a report.

Based on analysis of the data, the results of a study are included in the results section. The results of analysis of numerical data may be displayed using tables or graphs. Results based on qualitative data are summarized in a narrative description.

Interpretation of data is included in the discussion section of a report. Sometimes this section is titled results and discussion or discussion and conclusions. In this section the researcher applies knowledge gained by the study to previous research and current practices. Findings that are relevant to current clinical practices or theories may be included under the heading, conclusions and implications. Implications for further research also may be included under this heading.

BASIC RESEARCH CONCEPTS AND TERMS

Science is the search for knowledge. Ventry and Schiavetti (1986) described scientific method as a method of efficiently or methodically generating knowledge by recognizing a problem capable of objective study, collecting data by observation or experimentation, and drawing conclusions based on analysis of the data. Silverman (1993) further described scientific method as a set of rules used for describing, explaining, and predicting "events" that are observable and occur over time.

The scientific method is an effective tool for answering the type of questions it was designed to answer. However, as Siegel (1987) points out, some questions in communication disorders (e.g. those involving social and personal values and attitudes) cannot be answered using pure methods of science.

Basic and Applied Research

Theoretically, studies can be classified as basic or applied experimental research. *Basic research* focuses on answering important questions or deciphering the laws of nature (Hegde, 1994; Shearer, 1982). *Applied research* employs the answers to the basic questions to further research answers to practical problems such as questions involving clinical practice. Basic research provides a foundation for applied practical studies, and both types of research use experimental methods (Hegde, 1994; Shearer, 1982). There is little difference between applied and basic or experimental research (Hegde, 1994).

Basic research is often theoretical and designed to seek answers that explain phenomena and their causes and predict their appearance. Applied research seeks to answer practical questions. A foundation of basic research findings supports the continuation of applied study. Basic research is the foundation for research in rehabilitation (Findley & DeLisa, 1990). Shearer (1982) emphasized that combined basic and applied research projects probably make more significant contributions to the pool of knowledge in speech-language pathology and audiology. He further pointed out the importance of continued efforts involving answering the basic questions even though applied research tends to be perceived a more useful and practical expenditure of time and money. It is the combination of theory, research, and experience that provides a solid foundation of information in communication disorders (Siegel & Ingham, 1987). Doehring (1988) described the interaction between research and clinical practice. As a part of developing new clinical management strategies, new questions emerge for researchers to study. On the other hand, new findings based on research may result in the application of new clinical management practices.

Questions involving clinical management are answered using clinical or applied research models. Clinical research may be experimental or descriptive. Experimental studies involve use of a rigorous design in which variables are carefully controlled. Experimental research in speech-language pathology is often weakened somewhat statistically because some variables cannot be controlled (Shearer, 1982). For example, *ex post facto* (after the fact), or retrospective, experimental studies deal with something that happened earlier and cannot be controlled. For example, an individual who has a communication disorder has had numerous experiences associated with the disorder, which may vary from individual to individual. That person cannot be randomly selected for placement in the communication disordered group by the examiner. The person already has a communication disorder so an *ex post facto* condition placed the individual in that group, not a carefully controlled experimental procedure for randomizing experimental and control groups of subjects (Shearer, 1982).

Results of descriptive studies may involve nonstatistical means of reporting results. For example, results of attitude surveys are reported in descriptive terms. The research design for descriptive studies is not as rigorous as that for experimental studies.

Variables

Variables are capable of change or modification. They may vary in quality or quantity. Examples of qualitative variables might include the sex of an individual, the disorder of speech or language an individual has been diagnosed as having, or the type of clinical management selected for particular patients. Quantitative variables such as intelligence can be measured quantitatively or numerically. Discrete quantitative variables are not expressed in decimals nor fractions. Examples include the number of subjects in a study, scores on some tests, or the number of times a treatment is administered. Continuous variables can be expressed in any numerical value including fractions. Examples include age of subjects (i.e., 1.5 or $1\frac{1}{2}$ years), scores on some tests that allow results to be expressed in whole numbers or in fractions, or height and weight data describing subjects. Variables describe the population investigated by a study. Variables that do not change from individual to individual (such as a diagnosis of stuttering) are called constant variables.

Dependent Variables

Research in speech-language pathology and audiology is designed to investigate the causes of disorders and the effect(s) of various phenomena on behaviors associated with disorders of communication. Dependent variables are the effect of unknown etiology(ies). An example of a dependent variable is a hyperfunctional voice disorder characterized by a rough voice quality and accompanied by frequent upper respiratory infections, coughing, allergies, and laryngitis. As illustrated, the dependent variable must be described in operational terms so that it is clear how the variable will be identified and measured for a particular study (Hegde, 1994).

Independent Variables

Independent variables explain the dependent variables. For example, an individual's vocal habits (talking frequently, loudly, and with excessive laryngeal tension) along with behaviors associated with a medical condition (coughing, laryngitis) might constitute identified independent variables explaining the dependent variable, a voice disorder defined according to description and accompanying medical condition. By manipulating independent variables, an investigator may change dependent variables involving disorders of communication. For example, reducing abusive vocal habits and medically treating the laryngitis may successfully effect a change in voice characteristics to a smooth, more relaxed and pleasant voice production.

Hegde (1994) described three types of independent variables in communication disorders research: those that explain:

1. The cause of normal parameters of communication,
2. The development of abnormal communication, or
3. Identify treatment techniques that create optimal changes in communication.

The independent variables that can be manipulated (e.g., vocal habits and medical condition of the larynx and surrounding tissues) are *active variables* (Hegde, 1994). Some independent variables may be impossible to change (e.g., a predisposition for laryngeal vulnerability to abusive vocal habits). These are called *assigned variables* (Hegde, 1994). They may play a role in determining outcome but cannot be controlled by the investigator. The experimental researcher attempts to rule out assigned variables. For example, if patients identified as having a predisposition or vulnerability to some voice problems and those identified as less vulnerable both improve by changing voice habits and receiving medical intervention, the vulnerability variable may be ruled out or the assumption that it causes hyperfunctional phonation is at least reduced.

Control of Variables

Experiments generally involve the controlled manipulation of independent variable(s) in an effort to produce change in dependent variable(s). To determine specific cause-and-effect relationships, the experimenter must control other potential factors that might influence the outcome of the study. For example, an experimenter might attempt to show that abusive vocal habits cause hyperfunctional phonation by controlling for medical causes. Prior to conducting the experiment, the researcher might have all subjects examined and treated for medical conditions that might affect phonation. The experiment would then involve tracking both subjects' vocal habits and phonatory quality of their voices over a given period of time.

Hypotheses and Theories

Hypotheses are often formulated for the purpose of testing theories which explain a phenomenon, event, or condition. Questions may be stated in the form of a formal or working hypothesis. The formal or null hypothesis to be accepted or rejected by a study is stated in negative terms. A *null hypothesis* states that there is "no difference" or "no relationship" between groups or variables. For example, to test the theory that articulation errors may be caused by the presence of a hearing loss, a null hypothesis attempts to eliminate bias from the hypothesis by declaring no relationship between the variables (Hegde, 1994). Thus, the researcher attempts to reject the null hypothesis that there is no relationship between articulation development and the presence of a hearing loss. Hegde (1994) cautions, however, that the null hypothesis does not eliminate or control examiner bias. Objective interpretation of the results of a study requires objective, ethical research practices by a researcher with research education and experience, preferably initially in collaboration with experienced, objective researchers.

A working hypothesis also may simply ask a question: "Is there a difference" or "Is there a relationship" between groups or variables? Purpose statements are worded in many different ways. The reader will list examples of purpose statements and formal or working hypotheses while completing the exercises at the end of this chapter.

The acceptance or rejection of hypotheses based on the results of a research project are always interpreted as tentative. The findings of current studies may be replaced or expanded by future findings based on new theories, different clinical practice procedures, or changes in research methods. Like the records set by athletes, research findings often do not withstand expansion and changes in the knowledge base. As Silverman (1993, p. 13) stated: "The tentative nature of answers and hypotheses is due at least partially to the fact that observations are never complete. In other words, 'the data are never all in.' " Thus, the language used to convey the conclusions reached by a study revolves around the word "suggest" rather than "prove."

Validity and Reliability

When analyzing the accuracy of the results of a study, the investigator objectively attempts to answer questions of validity and reliability. When assessing the validity of a study, the primary question involves determining whether the information gathered actually contributes to answering the research question (Ventry & Schiavetti, 1986). For example, if the investigator identifies phonatory quality attributes using a Visipitch™ analysis with an inappropriate frequency range for some of the subjects, perturbation data might be questioned.

Hegde (1994) differentiates between the validity of the data defining the dependent variables and the validity of the experiment itself. Accuracy of the information about the phonation attributes of the subjects is an example of establishing the validity of data defining the dependent variable(s). The design of a study, including control methods for observing, collecting, and recording data and control of the variables that might have an impact on the outcome of the study, contributes to the validity of the experiment itself. For example, consistent tracking of relevant phonatory habits and phonatory attributes of all subjects would contribute to the validity of the experiment.

Both internal and external validity are important to establish when analyzing the results of a study. To establish internal validity, the experimenter determines if the experimental manipulation really made a difference (Kerlinger, 1973) by ensuring that extraneous factors that could influence the results are carefully controlled (Ventry & Schiavetti, 1986). To establish internal validity, the design of a study should effectively rule out all variables that might affect the dependent variable so that it can be concluded that the independent variable was ultimately responsible for any change in the dependent variable (Doehring, 1988). Hegde (1994) cites several factors that affect internal validity. Some of these are the effects of prior events, maturational changes in subjects, repeated testing, problems with instrumentation, bias in selection of subjects, and loss of subjects during the study, all of which could have the same effects on the dependent variable as the stated independent variable(s). In summary, internal validity involves answering the question of whether the experimental treatments actually made a difference in the study (Isaac & Michael, 1987).

For the voice study cited previously, internal validity could be established by demonstrating voice improvement using Visipitch™ data and a comparison of pre-and post-experiment perceptual analyses of the quality of the subjects' voices. Internal validity could be further established by reporting that: (1) the Visipitch™ equipment was properly set and calibrated, (2) subjects with phonatory disorders related to preexisting laryngeal conditions were not selected, (3) all perceptual judgments were made by the same speech-language pathologists whose perceptual judgments were calibrated to the same criteria in training sessions administered by the experimenter, (4) all subjects received the same training in identifying poor and establishing good vocal habits, and (5) all received the same medical diagnosis and treatment.

External validity is the extent to which the results of a study satisfy representativeness or generalizability (Kerlinger, 1973) or can be generalized to the population as a whole (Ventry & Schiavetti, 1986). Practical clinical use of findings is determined by establishing external validity. The extent to which effects of independent variables on dependent variables apply to the natural setting must be determined to establish external validity (Doehring, 1988). Hegde (1994) cites effects of treatment during a study and the knowledge of expected results by subjects as factors that may influence the external validity of a study. Isaac and Michael (1987) concluded that questions about external validity involving what populations, settings, treatment variables, and measurement variables to which an effect can be generalized may not be completely answerable. The researcher must attempt to control all variables as well as possible.

For the voice study, establishing external validity could be attempted by showing that: (1) the individuals selected for the study were typical in age, sex, and occupation to those generally reported in the literature as having chronic voice problems related to vocal abuse and/or inflammatory laryngeal conditions, (2) standard treatment information was given to all subjects about identification and reduction of vocal abuses, (3) typical medical management was used for the conditions diagnosed, and (4) establishing that the data provided by the Visipitch™ and pre- and post-perceptual analysis by examiners is typical of that collected by certified speech-language pathologists in varied clinical settings.

Three types of validity should be considered when using a test or questionnaire to measure an individual's knowledge or attitudes. These are content validity, criterion-related (including predictive and concurrent) validity, and construct validity. *Content validity* concerns whether the substance or content of a measure adequately represents the universe of content of the attribute being measured or how well the content of a test reflects the subject matter from which conclusions will be drawn (Isaac & Michael, 1987; Kerlinger, 1973). Kerlinger (1973) further explained that content validation is basically judgmental in that each item is judged for its pertinence or applicability to the property or characteristic being measured.

Ventry and Schiavetti (1986) further described content validity as a subjective means of logically explaining and evaluating test items to determine how well they reflect the characteristics to be measured. Content validity is concerned with adequately assessing all the aspects of the behaviors to be measured. For example, to assess IQ, the researcher usually assesses quantitative and verbal abilities because both have been shown to correlate with intelligence. For example, the content validity of a test of language development would be determined by identifying the important behaviors that reflect good or poor language performance, then determining whether the content of the test items reflects those behaviors or skills.

Ventry and Schiavetti (1986) define *criterion-related validity* as a test of whether a test (or measure) correlates with a known indicator (validating criterion) of the behavior (or characteristic) being measured. Two types of criterion-related validity include concurrent and predictive validity (Kerlinger, 1973). Kerlinger (1973) further described concurrent criterion-related validity as involving the ability to check a currently administered measuring instrument against an outcome occurring now. Predictive criterion-related validity involves the ability to check a measuring instrument against a future outcome. For example, future achievement is predicted by aptitude tests (predictive) and present (concurrent) and future (predictive) achievement are predicted by achievement tests. Present and future ability to learn and solve problems are predicted by IQ tests (Kerlinger, 1973). Thus, it is difficult to separate the predictive and concurrent components of criterion-related validity.

Criterion-related validity involves a test's ability to predict current or future performance. This may involve using correlation measures to compare test scores with criteria known to identify the same skills as the proposed test (Isaac & Michael, 1987). In fact, criterion-related data may be collected concurrently with the test to ascertain whether the test could replace the criteria-related procedure (Isaac & Michael, 1987). The major difficulty in establishing criterion-related validity is determining whether criteria exist to predict a specific skill or performance such as teaching effectiveness. The question of what constitutes appropriate criteria to measure teaching effectiveness has provided a hotbed of controversy for many years.

Construct validity involves scientific inquiry by testing a hypothesized relationship and validating a test and the theory behind it (Kerlinger, 1973). By investigating the qualities a test measures, the degree to which the concepts or theory behind the test account for performance on the test may be determined (Isaac & Michael, 1987). Thus, construct validity is concerned with the extent to which a testor questionnaire measures what it is supposed to measure by reflecting the theory, behavior, or characteristic to be measured (Ventry & Schiavetti, 1986). The scores on a test are correlated with other accepted measures of the same behavior. If subjects' scores on a new test are strongly correlated with their scores on an established test, then construct validity has been established.

Reliability refers to the consistency of a rater or of a measurement. Several words have been used to define reliability: dependability, predictability, consistency, credibility, and stability. In research, *reliability* refers to the consistency or correlation among repeated measures or observations. Reliability does not ensure accuracy or validity. Observations can be consistent without being accurate. For example, children's responses to audiometric screening in a noisy environment might very well be consistent but certainly would not be considered accurate or valid indicators of their hearing sensitivity.

Three types of reliability—intra-examiner (intra-rater or intra-judge), inter-examiner (inter-rater or inter-judge), and test-retest reliability should be assessed when establishing the reliability of the results of a study. Strong *intra-examiner reliability* infers that in repeated observations of the same subject the same examiner gets similar results. Intra-examiner reliability is usually not difficult to establish. However, *inter-examiner* reliability infers agreement among different observers measuring the same phenomenon. Inter-examiner reliability is considered a crucial measure of objectivity and is a necessary element to subjecting a study to scientific review (Hegde, 1994). *Test-retest reliability* involves how well subjects perform on one set of measurements as compared to their performance on a second evaluation of the same measurements.

Application of American Psychological Association standards for assessing the validity and reliability of well known scales for measuring disability, including communication and cognitive function of brain-injured patients, are discussed by Johnston, Findley, DeLuca, and Katz (1991). Because little is published about reliability and validity of scales in common clinical use, there is an enormous need for such studies.

Scales of Measurement

One important phase of a research project is the measurement of the appropriate variables. Scales of measurement provide a means of assigning numbers to events or objects according to prescribed rules. Preparing numerical data according to these rules allows the application of statistical treatment. Four scales or levels of measurement are used to categorize data. They are, in hierarchical order: nominal, ordinal, interval, and ratio scales.

Nominal Level of Measurement

The nominal (lowest) level of measurement classifies an event or object into a category. Examples include gender, name, medical chart number, stutterer or nonstutterer, individuals with and without a history of voice problems, hearing sensitivity (normal or abnormal), etiology of hearing loss (conductive or sensorineural), and language development (normal or abnormal). A subject is measured at this level by assigning the individual to one of the categories. Some variables at the nominal level are naturally measured as numerics (e.g., medical chart number); other variables are coded numerically (e.g., 1 = normal, 2 = abnormal). The numbers assigned denote differences and are not used mathematically for addition, subtraction, multiplication, or division. These functions would be meaningless at this level. Nonparametric procedures are used to identify changes in a group or differences between groups when assumptions for parametric procedures are not met (Ventry & Schiavetti, 1986). Thus, nonparametric statistics are appropriate treatment options when examining nominal data since nonparametric measures must be used if information cannot be derived at interval or ratio levels of measurement.

Ordinal Level of Measurement

The ordinal level of measurement shows the position of one variable relative to another. The intervals between variables are not equal. Examples of variables at the ordinal level include college classification (i. e., freshman, sophomore, junior, or senior), teaching ranks (i.e., instructor, assistant professor, associate professor, or professor), and severity of a disorder (i.e., mild, moderate, or severe). Examples of the ordinal categories for the variable, hearing sensitivity, include normal, mild, moderate, and severe. As with nominal level of measurement, variables at the ordinal level are frequently coded numerically (e. g., 1 = freshman, 2 = sophomore, 3 = junior, and 4 = senior). However, mathematical or numeric operations (addition, subtraction, multiplication, division) remain meaningless with ordinal measures. Nonparametric statistical methods are used to examine ordinal data.

Interval Level of Measurement

Interval scales are used when there are equal intervals between values but no absolute zero. For numeric operations to yield meaningful results, it is necessary to have equal intervals between adjacent numerical values. For example, the difference between 3 and 5 should be the same as the difference between 23 and 25. In both the interval and ratio levels of measurement, there are constant differences in data entries.

Examples of variables at the interval level include numerical ratings of vocal quality on a 5- or 7-point equal interval scale, numerical ratings reflecting stutterers' attitudes based on a 5-point Likert-type rating scale, standard or scaled scores on a language test, or IQ scores. Parametric statistics are used if the following criteria are met: (1) the subjects represent a "normal" population distribution; (2) the sample is sizable, usually more than 30; and (3) information is derived using the interval or ratio level of measurement (Ventry & Schiavetti, 1986). Thus, parametric statistical methods are used to examine equal interval data.

Ratio Level of Measurement

Ratio scales are interval scales with an absolute zero. In other words, it is assumed that the attribute being measured may not be present. This measure is more frequently appropriate for studies involving natural science than for studies in areas of social science. However, if the dependent variable is the frequency of events, such as frequency of moments of stuttering; has time measures, such as the latency period between seeing a printed word and saying it; involves a measured distance, such as measurement of the space constituting a velopharyngeal gap during phonation in patients with velopharyngeal incompetency; and so on, the ratio level may be appropriate. Height, weight, chronological age, hearing level in decibels, and fundamental frequency of a complex wave are additional examples of variables that can be measured at the ratio level.

The differences between interval and ratio measurements are that multiples are meaningful at the ratio level (a 6-mm velopharyngeal gap is twice as large as a 3-mm gap), and the units of the variables measured at the ratio level can be changed by simple multiplication (i.e., feet are converted into inches by multiplying by 12). These properties do not hold true for measurements at the interval level. For example, a person with an IQ of 100 is not twice as intelligent as someone with an IQ of 50. All numbers at the ratio level of measurement have mathematical properties, so parametric statistics are used to examine ratio interval data.

In summary, variables are treated either as categorical (e.g., gender, age, disorder) or quantitative (e.g., height, weight, IQ, frequency of occurrence). It is important that categories for variables be classified so that each subject fits into only one category. Quantitative variables usually are measured in discrete units (e.g., frequency, pounds, milliseconds, millimeters). These units must be carefully recorded as the data are collected.

Familiarity with basic research methods, concepts, and terms is vital to the preparation of the researcher/clinician in speech-language pathology. Kent (1989–1990) refers to a condition he calls fragmentation in outlook among new graduates in speech-language pathology. This condition leads to a narrow view of clinical assessment, research, education, and the structure of knowledge underlying clinical service and clinical science (Kent, 1989–1990). Such a narrow perspective prevents use of a holistic approach to research and clinical management which efficiently integrates what is known from all disciplines. Kamhi (1993) has pointed out the need for a stronger connection between research and clinical practice. Responsibility must be taken by both clinicians and researchers. Practitioners must have a functional understanding of theoretical bases underlying their clinical practices. Researchers must recognize that both qualitative and quantitative methods are capable of providing answers to important scientific and clinical questions (Duchan, 1994; Kamhi, 1994b; Plante, Kiernan, & Betts, 1994).

COLLABORATIVE RESEARCH

There are many advantages to collaborative research. Among them are: (1) generating ideas, (2) increasing efficiency, (3) improving overall quality of work, (4) sustaining motivation because collaboration entails a work commitment to others, (5) enhancing professional vitality, (6) facilitating options for professional development, (7) compensating for strengths and weaknesses, and (8) reducing stress and burnout as well as anxiety about research (Bayer & Smart, 1991; Doehring, 1988; Fox & Faver, 1984; Frank & Rickard, 1988; Ludlow, 1986; Pennebaker, 1991; Wylie & Fuller, 1985). On the other hand, there are also disadvantages to collaboration such as (1) the time required for negotiating and exchange; (2) long distance which incurs telephone, fax, mail, copying, and travel expenses; (3) the personal, socioemotional cost of developing and maintaining a working relationship with collaborators; (4) a slow or recalcitrant collaborator which can seriously delay or jeopardize a research project; and (5) determining authorship, that is, allocation of credit for research and writing (Fox & Faver, 1984).

Efficient communication among collaborators is critical because all team members should be consulted on major decisions (McFarlane & Hagler, 1993). Using couriers and faxes can be effective as can electronic mail and local area networking.

Typically, there are two types of collaborative efforts: informal and formal. Informal collaborators consist of technicians, friends, colleagues, and even casual acquaintances with special knowledge or experience

(Chial, 1985). These collaborators usually do not have specific responsibilities or time schedules. Formal collaboration involves an organized
group of reearchers who have agreed to certain responsibilities in the
completion of a project while meeting specified time lines for completing their obligations. Collaborators may be at the same institution or
at different institutions and geographically separated. It is important
to consider the role of the principle investigator in collaborative research as well as mentoring, because the latter is typically a beginning
researcher's first collaborative effort.

Role of the Principle Investigator

The roles and responsibilities of the principle investigator include: formulation of the research questions, project design, obtaining funding,
project start-up, and ongoing management, data analysis, and publication (Findley, Daum, & Stineman, 1990). Specific tasks are identified
in Table 3–2.

Mentoring

Mentoring is becoming increasingly important to professional development. Many professionals have had specific help before, during, and
after training from advisors or mentors (Bland & Schmitz, 1986). It is
generally recognized that mentoring has a positive effect on professional
development. Mentors or preceptors can help mentees avoid obstacles
of many kinds, provide professional support, develop contacts, and
provide insight into activities and benefits of professional organizations.
Studies in business, medicine, nursing, occupational therapy, ortho-
dontics and psychology have demonstrated the value of mentoring (Bland & Ruffin, 1992; Collins, 1983; Findley & DeLisa, 1990;
Jowers & Herr, 1990; Kirsling & Kochar, 1990; Rogers, Holloway, &
Miller, 1990; Silver, 1991; White, 1988; Williams & Blackburn, 1988).
Mentoring has recently received attention from the American Speech-
Language-Hearing Association (ASHA 1989a, 1989b, 1989c). The purpose of this section is to: (1) explain the importance of mentoring to mentees and mentors, (2) clarify erroneous assumptions
about mentoring, (3) describe how to select a mentor, and (4) review
mentoring activity in speech-language pathology and audiology.

Importance of Mentoring

Academic training alone is not sufficient preparation to function as a professional (Ainsworth et al., 1972). According to Slater (1993) "mentors

TABLE 3-2. Tasks of the Principal Investigator

Formulation of the Question
Initiate research content area
Formulate hypothesis
Review the literature*
Contact outside experts

Project Design
Outline project proposal and seek review*
Select collaborators, consultants, and equipment*
Obtain funding
Make inquiries to potential funding sources*
Calculate budget including salaries, equipment, and supplies*
Write project proposals in format of funding agent*

Project Start-up
Initiate formal institutional review
Design data forms*
Obtain equipment
Designate or hire staff

Ongoing Project Management
Recruit subjects
Review rate of recruitment
Enforce recruitment of subjects
Conduct pilot studies
Collect, enter, reduce data
Conduct research staff meetings at regular intervals

Project Analysis
Chose statistical tests*
Review data
Analyze data*
Interpret data

Publication
Prepare manuscript*
Edit manuscript*
Present research results at conferences

Source: From "Research in Physical Medicine and Rehabilitation: The Role of the Principal Investigator" by T. W. Findley, M. C. Daum, and G. Stineman, 1990, *American Journal of Physical Medicine and Rehabilitation, 90,* p. 40, with permission. Copyright 1990 by Williams & Wilkins.
*Portions of these tasks may be delegated to collaborators and/or consultants

often provide an education that is not taught in the classroom" (p. 55). Most productive professionals have had help from mentors or advisors (Bland & Schmitz, 1986). Naas and Flahire (1991) believe that mentoring "describes many preprofessionals' only relationships where there is a commitment to extending the educational process beyond the lecture hall" (p. 40). Mentoring can help new professionals set priorities improve their skills, and survive the politics of professional life (Irby, 1993).

Mentors have been described as advocates, critics, facilitators, protectors, supporters, teachers, tutors, counselors, preceptors, role models, guides, mother surrogates, and best friends (Davis & Parker, 1979; Jowers & Herr, 1990; Redland, 1989; Sands, Parson, & Duane, 1991). A mentor may fulfill a number of functions, but it is an unusual mentor who can fulfill all these functions (Rogers, Holloway, & Miller, 1990). Perhaps the most important function of a mentor is teaching the mentee professional behavior (Bernstein & Rozen, 1989). In a survey of 2,010 biomedical trainees, Kalichman and Friedman (1992) found that the majority had received training in research ethics from their mentors. Table 3–3 contains a list of mentor functions developed by Strange and Hekelman (1990). The relative importance of these functions varies and may change over time. Also different mentors may be needed at different career stages and ages.

Mentors also benefit from the mentoring process. Among the benefits to mentors are professional rejuvenation, exchange of ideas with the mentee, collaborative research, and a personal sense of satisfaction from sharing with colleagues (Strange & Hekelman). Moore (1982) suggested mentoring also can help ensure continuity and facilitate the mentor's maintaining power and influence.

Erroneous Assumptions About Mentoring

There are several questionable assumptions and half-truths about mentoring that can adversely affect selection of a mentor (see Table 3–4). Students and neophyte professionals can select more appropriate mentors if they know the truths behind these questionable assumptions and half-truths and how to avoid problem mentors.

Selecting a Mentor

Not all audiologists and speech-language pathologists are qualified by disposition, knowledge, experience, or productivity to be mentors. Unfortunately, there are problem mentors, such as "Park Bench" mentors, who are unproductive sentimentalists, and "Bumbling" mentors,

TABLE 3–3. Types of Mentoring

Mentor's Role	Examples
Advocate	Fostering credibility Sponsorship
Nurturer	Career planning Collegiality Counseling Encouraging the dream Generating enthusiasm and confidence Providing moral support Reality testing Serving as a sounding board
Friend in the professional setting	Broadening perspectives Developing role clarity Providing access to key people and resources Understanding the professional environment
Role model	Intellectual stimulation Involving the mentee in one of the mentor's projects Teaching by example
Teacher	Coaching Constructive feedback Developing specific knowledge or skills Taskmaster

Source: From "Mentoring Needs and Family Medicine Faculty" by K. Strange and F. Hekelman, 1990, Family Medicine, 22, 183–185, with permission. Copyright 1990 by Family Medicine.

who give poor advice (Bell, 1984). Another mentoring problem is related to the "bad halo" effect in which the ineffectiveness or unpopularity of a mentor adversely affects the mentee and hinders rather than helps professional development (Loftin, 1987).

Selecting a mentor is both important and difficult. It is important because the success and quality of one's initial experience with conducting research depends on the mentoring skills of the person selected.

TABLE 3–4. Questionable and Correct Assumptions about Mentoring

Questionable Assumptions	Correct Assumptions
Mentoring is a formal, long-term arrangement.	Mentoring can be an informal luncheon, a telephone call, or several meetings over time.
Men are mentors but not women.	Women can serve as mentors for men or other women.
An individual should have only one mentor at a time.	An individual might have one mentor in one area and a different mentor for another.
A mentor must be older, have more training, and years of professional experience.	A mentor only has to be more knowledgeable in a particular area.
An individual can only be a mentor or a mentee.	An individual may be both a mentor and a mentee.
Researchers need mentors, but clinicians and academicians do not.	All professionals need mentors.
Selecting a mentor or a mentee is an unimportant decision.	Selecting a mentor or mentee is an important decision requiring careful consideration.
Mentors do not benefit from the mentoring process.	Mentors benefit from the mentoring process.
Mentors and mentees should be a homogenous group.	Mentors and mentees may represent a heterogenous group (men and women varied in age, interests, experience, and skills).
It is unnecessary to prepare professionals for the mentor role.	It is necessary to prepare professionals to be mentors.

It is difficult because the decision is based on special needs and de-
sires that may be difficult to identify early in one's career. On the other
hand, at mid-career one may need a different kind of mentor (Friel-
Patti, 1993; Jenuchim & Shapiro, 1992).

Mentors should be selected on the basis of an objective analysis
of data rather than the usual method based on hearsay and reputation
(Collins, 1983; Lanks, 1990; Nemko, 1988). Several factors should be
considered in selecting a mentor. These factors include individual learning needs, area(s) of specialization, availability of a mentor, a mentor's
clinical experience, recent scholarly productivity, assigned research
space, percent of time allocated for research, and productivity of the
mentor's mentees. Scholarly productivity can be considered relative to
quantitative, qualitative, peer judgment, and eminence or prestige measures as shown in Table 3–5. Furthermore, the mentor should have
promoted the careers of others, particularly of his or her mentees. Lanks
(1990) believes the ability to place students in professional positions
is the ultimate test of a mentor. The mentor's mentees should also be
evaluated relative to such factors as professional affiliation(s) and productivity. Research productivity of mentors and their mentees can be
evaluated simultaneously by computerized reference searches.

Mentoring Activity in Speech-Language Pathology and Audiology

ASHA's 1992 Omnibus Survey (Slater, 1992) included several findings
about mentoring. The results indicated: (1) only 36.2% of the respondents had a mentor; (2) respondents who had not had a mentor were
almost equally divided when asked if they wished they had; (3) slightly
more than one third of the respondents (35.6%) had served as a mentor; (4) of those who had been a mentor, 75% served as mentor for
someone of the same gender, and a few (18.6%) mentored more than
one individual; (5) more respondents with doctoral degrees (42.3%) had
a mentor than those with master's degrees (36.1%); and (6) almost 60%
of doctoral degree respondents had been mentors compared to 34.2%
of respondents with master's degrees. Apparently opinions about mentoring are mixed, and speech-language pathologists and audiologists
with doctoral degrees are more likely to have been mentees or mentors, although Gavett (1987) emphasized the importance of mentoring
for clinical supervisors with master's degrees.

The relatively low prevalence of mentoring found in the ASHA
Omnibus Survey (Slater, 1992) may be related to gender and differences among employment settings. The vast majority of ASHA members are female (ASHA, 1990b). In predominately female professions,

TABLE 3–5. Measures of Productivity

Quantitative Measures	Qualitative Measures
Number of pages published	Articles in quality journals
Number of publications	Citations of published materials
Number of papers presented at professional meetings	Citations of presentations in published materials
Grants submitted	Grants received
Peer Judgment	**Eminence Measures**
Peers at institution	Grant review committees
Peers with publications training	Reviewer or editor of peer-reviewed journal(s)
Peers at other institutions	Honors or awards from profession
Self-evaluation	Officer of national professional associations
Departmental chairs	Invited papers and guest lectures
Deans	Number of dissertations supervised

Sources: "Research in Physical Medicine and Rehabilitation: XI. Research training setting the stage for lifelong learning" by T. W. Findley and J. A. DeLisa, 1990, *American Journal of Physical Medicine and Rehabilitation, 69,* 323–329; *Evaluating Faculty for Promotion and Tenure* by R. Miller, 1987, San Francisco: Jossey-Bass; and "Using Faculty Research Performance for Academic Quality Rankings" by D. Webster and C. Conrad, 1986, *New Directions for Institutional Research, 50,* 43–57.

females often do not have opportunities for mentoring (DeAngelis, 1991; Sands, Parson, & Duane, 1991). This may be due in part to a lack of available mentors for women because there are fewer women in leadership positions. Mentors usually hold high positions and professional status (Berryman-Fink, 1989). Difficulties with cross-gender mentoring (males mentoring females) have been reported due to perceived reinforcement of stereotypical roles of male power and female dependence, issues of intimacy and sexuality that sometimes occur in cross-gender mentor relationships, and resentment from co-workers, spouses and family (Berryman-Fink, 1989). ASHA's (1991a) report on gender-related issues indicated that women need mentorship experiences, to know how to select appropriate mentors, and the "value in having a variety of role models/mentors who may even include male mentors" (p. 6).

Mentoring appears to be more common in academic settings. For example, Sands, Parson, and Duane (1991) found that the majority of faculty at a public university had a mentor. Only a small percentage of speech-language pathologists (5%) and audiologists (8%) are employed in a college or university (Slater, 1992). Furthermore, there is a gender difference between employment settings. More males in ASHA (15%) are employed in a college or university than females (2.7%) (Shewan, 1988).

Few speech-language pathologists and audiologists have or have had mentors (Slater, 1992). There are, however, some personal accounts of mentoring in the speech-language pathology and audiology literature (Ashmore, 1992; Butler, 1992; Friel-Patti, 1992; Seymour, 1992; Stephens, 1991; Stewart, 1992; Tibbits, 1992). This is an encouraging trend due to the relative paucity of female mentors reported in speech-language pathology and other professions. In several accounts, the author has been both a mentee and mentor (Ashmore, 1992; Butler, 1992; Seymour, 1992; Stephens, 1991). Perhaps those who have been mentees are more likely to be aware of the value of mentoring. Also, cross-gender mentoring, for example, a male mentee with a female mentor has been reported (Tibbits, 1992). Some of the mentees reported having more than one mentor, and most mentees and mentors had doctoral degrees.

Mentoring programs have been described by several organizations, including ASHA, three state speech-language-hearing associations, and several speech-language and hearing facilities. ASHA is developing a mentorship program to provide beginning researchers the opportunity to work with senior researchers (ASHA, 1989a, 1989b, 1989c; Shewan, 1989, 1990a, 1990b). ASHA has also provided guidelines for starting a mentoring program (Gelatt, 1992). Colorado (Kovach & Moore, 1992), Florida (Rosenberg, 1992), and Texas (Breeding, 1992; Friel-Patti, 1991) have all established mentorship programs within their state speech-language-hearing associations. Such programs also have been established in different facilities. For example, the Veterans Administration (VA) held a national workshop on mentoring for their speech-language pathologists and audiologists (Wofford, Boysen, & Riding, 1991), and the Richardson, Texas, school speech-language therapy program has developed a mentorship program (Duncan, 1992).

THE RESEARCH PROCESS

By the time a research project is published, it has been organized and presented in an established, straightforward format. However, the actual process of doing research is not as organized as one might think after reading numerous published articles that have been repeatedly edited. Hegde (1994) described a formative view of research as an evolving process. After much discussion and pondering, numerous false starts, and repeated attempts, a project may emerge and develop. Many worthy projects are abandoned in the process. For assistance in finishing a well-organized, comprehensive project following the disorder and confusion that sometimes accompanies the process, Braddom (1990) provides an in-depth outline or guide to assist in identification of specific omissions or errors in the major sections of a completed research project.

Some significant findings in science over the years have been based on accidental discoveries. Hegde (1994) refers to serendipity in research as evidence that worthwhile projects are not always carefully planned. Accidental discoveries may be the reward for flexibility and a creative sense of inquiry on the part of observers when conducting a research project.

COMMON MYTHS ABOUT RESEARCH AND HOW TO AVOID THEM

Several myths about research in speech-language pathology and audiology have been carried over from previous decades. Other erroneous concepts about the research process are of more recent origin, and are sometimes supported by professionals who are well-intentioned but feel strongly that what they believe is true. This "solid conviction" approach results in strongly stated opinions. Heard loudly and frequently enough, these opinions can be misinterpreted as "facts" by the inexperienced researcher. Students and practicing clinicians will be more productive researchers if they are familiar with the truths behind these myths (see Figure 3–1). The myths and the truths behind them are identified in Table 3–6.

SUMMARY

Research is a procedure for following rules for asking and answering questions. The research process requires that the researcher develop a command of basic research terminology and become knowledgeable

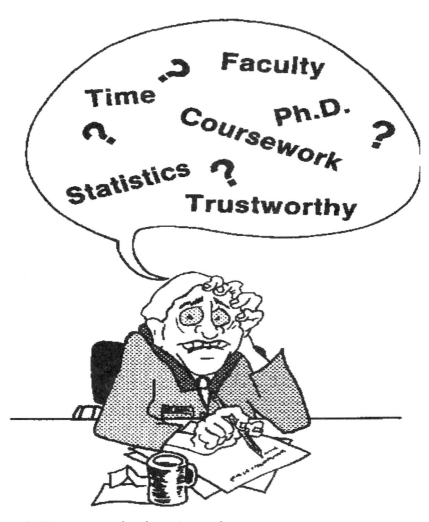

FIGURE 3–1. Myths about Research.

about the scientific method. There is little room for arrogance in the research process. One must understand the level of importance of a study in comparison to the universe of knowledge on the topic. Furthermore, the quest for absolute proof or conclusive findings is incompatible with scientific method. All findings are considered tentative until the next piece of the puzzle is supplied in follow-up studies.

There is a need for a stronger connection between researchers and clinicians in speech-language pathology. Responsibility for forming this

TABLE 3–6. Myths and Truths About Research

Myth	Truth	References
Academic course work prepares one to do research.	Academic course work often does not prepare one to do research.	Bardach and Kelley (1991) Coney and Burk (1987) Kent (1983)
Research is too time consuming.	Research need not be particularly time consuming.	Boice (1989) Silverman (1985)
Clinical practice and research activities are different.	Clinical practice and research are similar; they both use scientific methodology.	Connell and McReynolds (1988) Drew and Hardman (1985) Findley (1989) Findley and DeLisa (1990) Kamhi (1984) Ringel (1972)
The doctorate is necessary to do research.	Research is done by individuals without a doctorate.	Pannbacker, Lass, & Middleton (1988) Silverman (1993)
Extensive knowledge of statistics is essential.	Research is more than statistics.	Drew and Hardman (1985) Leedy (1989) Shearer (1982) Silverman (1993) Ventry and Schiavetti (1986)

(continued)

TABLE 3-6. (continued)

Myth	Truth	References
Published information is reliable.	Some published information is unreliable.	Bordens and Abbott (1988) Ventry and Schiavetti (1986) Woodford (1967)
Selecting a faculty research advisor is an unimportant decision.	Selecting a research advisor is an important decision requiring careful consideration.	Chial (1985) Davis and Parker (1979) Hegde (1994) Neumann and Finaly-Neuhaus (1991)
Experienced researchers are above criticism.	Experienced researchers are subjected to criticism throughout the research process.	Deep and Sussman (1990) Doehring (1988) Luey (1987) Ogden (1991) O'Connor and Woodford (1977) Troyka (1990)
Reasons for doing research do not apply to me.	Reasons for doing research apply to all speech-language pathologists and audiologists.	Adams et al. (1984) Braxton (1991) Chial (1985) Davis and Parker (1979) Findley and DeLisa (1990) Hegde (1994) Hunter and Kuh (1987) Shprintzen (1991)

I cannot do research; I don't know where to start.	There are strategies designed to facilitate research productivity.	Boice (1989) Deep and Sussman (1990) Pannbacker, Lass, & Middleton (1988)
Research is not an ethical responsibility.	Speech-language pathologists and audiologists have an ethical responsibility to do research.	ASHA (1991b) Frye (1991)
Research is only for students.	Research is for students and practicing professionals.	Horowitz (1988)
Research is dull.	Research is exciting.	Horowitz (1988)
Time management is unimportant to research.	Time management is vital to research.	Boice (1989)
Socialization is not related to research productivity.	Socialization is related to research productivity.	Bland and Schmitz (1986)
Publish or perish is untrue.	Publish or perish is an academic truth.	Boice (1989) Boyes et al. (1984)

(continued)

TABLE 3-6. *(continued)*

Myth	Truth	References
Most practicing professionals do research.	Very few professionals do research.	Boice and Jones (1984) Chial (1985) Kraemer and Lyons (1989) Mansour and Punch (1984)
Early research productivity is unrelated to later research productivity.	Early research is related to later research productivity.	Allison and Stewart (1974) Frank and Rickard (1988)
Productive researchers work on one research project at a time.	Productive researchers work on several projects simultaneously.	Bland and Schmitz (1986)

connection must be assumed by both clinicians and researchers. In a behavioral science such as speech-language pathology both qualitative and quantitative methods can provide answers to scientific and clinical questions.

Informal and formal collaborative research efforts are effective means of increasing research productivity and creativity. For the novice researcher, the opportunity to work with an experienced researcher is an effective means of getting started. Mentoring is a mutually beneficial process. Like the giving of gifts, it is rewarding to share knowledge and expertise. In addition, the effective mentor provides the apprentice with the truths behind the myths about research.

STUDY EXERCISES

1. Review the article you selected to comment, praise, and/or condemn in a letter to the editor for Exercise 2 in Chapter 2. This article is on a topic that you selected in Exercise 4 in Chapter 1. If you would prefer to use a different article for this activity on the topic referenced as part of Exercise 4 in Chapter 1, feel free to do so. Use a word processor to provide the information requested on the article as follows. Use the exact format provided. Provide requested information verbatim from the article when appropriate.

Title:

Author(s):

Problem Statement:

Statement included in the literature review that provides a reason for further investigation:

How many studies were cited in the literature review?

Purpose of the Study:

Research Question(s) or Hypothesis(es):

Type of research design:

Summarize the procedure used in doing the study:

Include a description of and number of subjects, how they were selected, independent and dependent variables, data analysis includng specific statistical application, type of statistics used, and type of study (basic or applied, experimental or descriptive, group or single subject).

How did the author(s) display the results of the study?

Briefly summarize the interpretation of the data in the discussion section.

How did the researcher(s) compare the findings of this study with findings of previous studies cited in the literature review?

What implications for future research on the topic were provided?

How did the author(s) word the conclusion(s) of the study?

2. Analyze the use of scientific method in the article you selected for Exercise 1 above.

Was the problem clearly stated?

Determine intersubjective testability by analyzing the procedure and concluding whether the study would be easily duplicated by you or another researcher.

Evaluate the reliability of the study by studying the number of observations or subjects used and means of calculating the reliability information.

Analyze the organization of the findings. Were the tables, figures, or graphs clear and easily interpreted by the reader? Was the information presented logically and in an organized format?

Did the findings support the stated conclusions?

How was validity established?

3. What is your impression of the study reviewed in Exercises 1 and 2? Include in your discussion your perception of the importance of the findings on the available pool of knowledge on the topic, the apparent knowledge of the researchers on the topic under investigation, and the application of scientific method. Can you think of any additional implications of the study or additional areas for research generated by the study but not stated by the investigators?

4. How is the word "measurement" used in research and statistics?

5. List and define the four levels of measurement and give an example of each level.

6. What is necessary to have numeric operations yield meaningful results? Which level(s) of measurement has/have this property?

7. The property of multiplication is meaningful at what level(s) of measurement?

8. Define validity and name and explain the different types of validity with examples of each.

9. Define reliability and name and explain the different types of reliability?

10. What are the advantages and disadvantages of collaborative research? Would you rather do research alone or as part of a team using a collaborative model? Explain your answer.

11. You have decided that in order to develop professionally, you need a mentor. Whom would you pick and why?

12. You have decided to organize a research team as its lead investigator. Proceed with your plans by answering the following questions.

    a. What will you include in a list of things to consider when establishing a research team?

    b. What will be your responsibilities as the principle investigator of your team?

    c. As a researcher, what skills do you feel you have that will contribute most effectively to the team's efforts?

    d. As a researcher, what skills do you feel you need to develop to more effectively contribute to the team's efforts?

13. What type of research is conducted by most speech-language pathologists and audiologists? Is this type of research conducive to the collaborative research model?

14. How might one proceed in developing a research network?

15. Are research and clinical service mutually exclusive? As part of your answer describe the relationship between research and clinical service.

SUGGESTED READINGS

Ashmore, L. (1992). Reflections on mentoring. *Communicologist, 17*(1), 9–10.

Doehring, D. G. (1988). *Research strategies in human communication disorders.* Boston, MA: College-Hill Press., Chapter 2, The sequence of events in research, 9–22.

Gelatt, J. P. (1992). Starting a mentoring program. *Asha, 29*(5), 48.

Hegde, M. N. (1994). *Clinical research in communicative disorders: Principles and strategies.* Austin, TX: Pro-Ed., Chapter 1, Why study science and research methods?, 3–20.

Silverman, F. H. (1993). *Research design and evaluation in speech-language pathology and audiology.* Englewood Cliffs, NJ: Prentice-Hall, Chapter 3, Research as a process of asking and answering questions, 22–40.

C H A P T E R   4

TYPES OF RESEARCH

MARY H. PANNBACKER AND GRACE F. MIDDLETON

- Experimental Research
- Quasi-Experimental Research
- Nonexperimental Research
- Other Types of Research
- Summary
- Study Exercises
- Suggested Readings

Classification of research into specific categories is not easy because there are a number of different research strategies. There is also lack of agreement about these categories as well as overlap among the various types of research so that a specific research project may fit more than one of the classifications (Ventry & Schiavetti, 1986). Furthermore, different research activities use different methods, depending on the purposes of the study, the nature of the problem and the alternatives appropriate for its investigation (Hegde, 1994; Isaac & Michael, 1987). Hegde (1994) warns that "within their limitations, all types of research contribute something to the knowledge base. Some types of research, however, do more than others in helping us understand the events we study" (p. 103). Research can be classified as: experimental, non-experimental and quasi-experimental. Other types of research include case studies, evaluation research, field studies, historical research, needs assessments, pilot studies, secondary analysis, and survey research. Table 4–1 presents examples of the different types of research in speech-language pathology and audiology that are discussed inthis chapter.

EXPERIMENTAL RESEARCH

In experimental research, the independent variable is controlled to measure its effect on the dependent variables (Shearer, 1982). In other words, experimental research is used to examine possible cause-and-effect-relationships by exposing one or more experimental groups to one or more conditions and comparing the results to one or more control groups (Isaac & Michael, 1987). This type of research has also been referred to as the cause-and-effect method, the pretest-posttest control group design, and the laboratory method (Leedy, 1989). The distinguishing feature of experimental research is the experiment and control of the main variables; other types of research do not involve an experiment (Hegde, 1994; Shearer, 1982). Experimental research is considered by many to be the best or most powerful research design, but it is not the only acceptable type of research (Hegde, 1994; Ottenbacher, 1990; Polit & Hungler, 1991). Shearer (1982) points out that the most appropriate type "of research is the one that best fits the problem and the situation available" (p. 10).

The three characteristics of experimental research described by Polit and Hungler (1991) were: (1) "manipulation — the experimenter does something to at least some of the subjects in the study; (2) control — the experimenter introduces one or more controls over the experimental situation, including the use of a control group; and

TABLE 4–1. Examples of Types of Research in Speech-Language Pathology and Audiology

Purpose	Types of Research	Authors
Determine if noise level in a high school woodwork class contributes to the incidence of hearing loss.	Experimental	Lankford and West (1993)
Compare speech and language comprehension and production between very low birth weight and normal birth weight 8-year-olds.	Descriptive, ex post facto	Aram and associates (1991)
Follow hearing aid users for 1 year post fitting.	Descriptive, longitudinal	Bentley and associates (1993)
Language acquisition after mutism, a longitudinal study.	Descriptive, longitudinal	Windsor, Doyle, and Siegel (1994)
Test the general question of whether the focus construct is statistically significant in predicting intervention outcome.	Ex post facto	Kwiatkowski and Shriberg (1993)

(continued)

TABLE 4-1. (continued)

Purpose	Types of Research	Authors
Describe the occurrence of laryngeal pathologies and their distribution across age, sex, and occupation in a group seeking physician treatment.	Ex post facto	Herrington-Hall and associates (1988)
Speech deterioration in amyotrophic lateral sclerosis.	Case study	Kent and associates (1991)
Language acquisition after mutism.	Case study, longitudinal	Windsor, Doyle, and Siegel (1994)
Demonstrate how the maximum likelihood procedure can be used for analysis of group and individual data in aphasia research.	Case study, group design	Bates, McDonald, MacWhinney, and Applebaum (1991)
Reanalysis of data from previous study.	Secondary analysis	Bates, Applebaum, and Allaid (1991)

Consumer satisfaction for assessing quality of services.	Evaluation research	Rao and associates (1992)
How voice quality can be most appropriately assessed, what reasonable standards for intra- and interrater reliability of perceptual judgments might be, and how reliability of ratings and levels of agreement within and among listeners might be maximized.	Historical	Kreiman and associates (1993)
Interpreting results of studies comparing fluent speech characteristics of stutterers and nonstutterers.	Historical	Armson and Kalinowski (1994)
Review of currently available preschool speech-language screening tests.	Historical	Sturner and associates (1994)
Nonlinear phonology.	Historical	Bernhardt and Stoel-Gammon (1994)

(continued)

TABLE 4–1. (continued)

Purpose	Types of Research	Authors
Investigate speech-language pathologists' perceptions of administrative and nonadministrative support.	Pilot; survey (telephone)	Schetz and Billingsley (1990)
Obtain information about speech and hearing professionals' knowledge of basic genetic counseling.	Pilot; survey (mail)	Chermak and Wagner-Bitz (1993)
Efficacy of speech-language therapy for aphasia.	Meta-analysis	Whurr, Lorch, and Nye (1992)

(3) randomization—the experimenter assigns subjects to a control or experimental group on a random basis" (p. 152).

Procedures of Experimental Research

Isaac and Michael (1987) have outlined the steps in experimental research (see Table 4–2). This outline is useful in understanding experimental research and knowing the procedures that a researcher might utilize.

Strengths and Weaknesses of Experimental Research

According to Hegde (1994) "the strengths of experimental research are the strengths of science itself" (p. 95). It is the most appropriate method

TABLE 4–2. Seven Steps in Experimental Research

1. Survey the literature relating to the problem.
2. Identify and define the problem.
3. Formulate a problem hypothesis, deducing the consequences and defining basic terms and variables.
4. Construct an experimental plan:
   a. Identify all nonexperimental variables that might contaminate the experiment, and determine how to control them.
   b. Select a research design.
   c. Select a sample of subjects to represent a given population, assign subjects to groups, and assign experimental treatments to groups.
   d. Select or construct and validate instruments to measure the outcome of the experiment.
   e. Outline procedures for collecting the data, and possibly conduct a pilot or "trial run" test to perfect the instruments or design.
   f. State the statistical or null hypothesis.
5. Conduct the experiments.
6. Reduce the raw data in a manner that will produce the best appraisal of the effect which is presumed to exist.
7. Apply an appropriate test of significance to determine the confidence one can place on the results of the study.

Source: From *Understanding Educational Research* by D. B. Van Dalen and W. J. Meyer, 1966 (Rev.). New York: McGraw-Hill, with permission. Copyright 1966 McGraw-Hill.

for testing hypotheses of cause-and-effect relationships between variables. Experimental research offers greater corroboration than any other type of research in that if the independent variable is manipulated in a certain way, then certain consequences in the dependent variable may be expected to ensue.

Experimental research has several weaknesses. First, there are many situations in which experimental research cannot be conducted because of ethical or practical considerations (Polit & Hungler, 1991). Another problem with experimental research is the Hawthorne effect. This refers to the effect on the dependent variable caused by changes in subjects' behavior because they know they are participating in a study (Huck, Cormier, & Bounds, 1974; Polit & Hungler, 1991; Ventry & Schiavetti, 1986). Despite the problems inherent in experimental research, Hegde (1994) believes none of the "weaknesses of experimental research seem to be valid" (p. 94).

QUASI-EXPERIMENTAL RESEARCH

Variations of "true" experimental research are considered quasi-experimental because they do not have the same degree of experimental control or inferential confidence (Ottenbacher, 1990). This type of research is sometimes referred to as pseudoexperimental or pre-experimental (Huck et al., 1974). Quasi-experimental research, like experimental research, involves manipulation of an independent variable but does not have a comparison group or randomization (Polit & Hungler, 1991). The two characteristics of quasi-experimental research identified by Isaac and Michael (1987) are: "(1) quasi-experimental typically involves applied settings where it is not possible to control all the relevant variables but only some of them; and (2) the distinction between true and quasi-experimental research is tenuous, particularly where human subjects are involved" (p. 54). The steps in quasi-experimental research are similar to those used in experimental research which are outlined in Table 4–2. Quasi-experimental research, however, unlike experimental research, does not allow inferences about cause-and-effect relationships.

NONEXPERIMENTAL RESEARCH

Nonexperimental research can be categorized as either (1) descriptive or (2) *ex post facto*. There is, however, overlap between these categories; many have similar characteristics making it difficult to distinguish between categories. Also there is little agreement about terminology (see

Figure 4–1). For example, what is developmental research to one researcher may be correlational research to another.

Descriptive Research

Descriptive research is designed to systematically describe situations or events as they naturally occur, in other words, the status of phenomena of interest as they currently exist (Polit & Hungler, 1991). It is a type of research in which the distribution of selected dependent variables is observed and recorded (Hegde, 1994). Descriptive research is used to study group differences, developmental trends, and relationships among variables (Ventry & Schiavetti, 1986). Sometimes this type of research is called normative or developmental research (Hegde, 1994). Developmental research which focuses on changes over time may be: cross-sectional, longitudinal and semi-longitudinal (Shearer, 1982; Ventry & Schiavetti, 1986). Not all such research is developmental in the maturational sense; it may be designed, for example, to study the course of progressive pathology.

Cross-sectional research involves selecting subjects from various age groups and observing differences between the behaviors or characteristics of the groups. This approach has several advantages: (1) it is less costly and less time consuming than longitudinal research, and

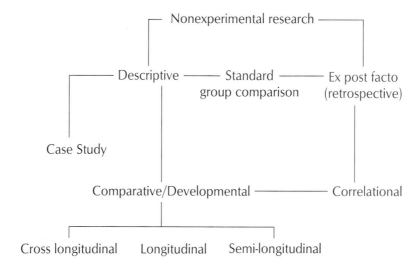

FIGURE 4–1. Classification of Nonexperimental Research.

(2) it is relatively immune to subject attrition. The greatest disadvantage is the possibility that results could be attributable to biased selection of the cross-sectional groups. There are a variety of terms used for cross-sectional research: disease frequency, survey, and prevalence study (Rosenfeld, 1991).

Many consider longitudinal research stronger than cross-sectional research because the same group of subjects is followed over time. This approach has the disadvantages of being expensive, time consuming, and vulnerable to subject attrition. Because of these problems, only a small number of subjects can be studied. Synonyms for longitudinal research include cohort study, follow-up study, incidence study, and perspective study (Rosenfeld, 1991).

The semi-longitudinal approach is a compromise designed to maximize the strengths and minimize the weaknesses of the cross-sectional and longitudinal approaches. This involves dividing the total age span to be studied into several overlapping age spans, selecting subjects whose ages are at the lower edge of each new age span, and following them until they reach the upper age of the span (Shearer, 1982; Ventry & Schiavetti, 1986).

The descriptive approach has limitations. First, unlike experimental research, descriptive research does not lead to cause-and-effect conclusions. The description of relationships among variables or of differences between groups does not provide sufficient information for making cause-and-effect statements. Second, but related, descriptive research is considered by some to be inferior to experimental research. Ventry and Schiavetti (1986) believe that descriptive research is not an inferior method because there are situations in which it is more appropriate and situations in which experimental research is more appropriate.

Ex Post Facto Research

Ex post facto, or after the fact, research is research "conducted after the variations in the independent variable have occurred in the natural course of events" (Polit & Hungler, 1991, p. 176). It is not experimental or quasi-experimental because it lacks active manipulation of the independent variable and does not result in cause-and-effect conclusions. Ex post facto research is also referred to as case control study, case history study, correlational research, and trohoc study (Rosenfeld, 1991).

The primary strength of ex post facto research is that it is a method of collecting data in research situations that do not lend themselves to experimental inquiry. Kerlinger (1973) identified three major limitations of ex post facto research: "(1) the inability to manipulate independent variables, (2) the lack of power to randomize, and (3) the risk of improper interpretation" (p. 390).

Existing clinical data found in client records are used for ex post facto or retrospective studies. Findley and Daum (1989) provided guidelines for design and execution of research projects using existing clinical data. Potential difficulties and limitations can be identified by: (1) review of published studies; (2) use of clinical experience, and (3) review of individual client records.

Reasons for Conducting Nonexperimental Research

Nonexperimental research is conducted for several reasons. First, a number of independent variables associated with individuals and institutions are not amenable to control and randomization. Second, numerous variables that could be controlled experimentally should not be for ethical reasons. Third, it may not be possible or practical to manipulate variables, that is, to conduct a true experiment because of insufficient time, inconvenience to clients or staff, lack of administrative support, or inadequate funding (Polit & Hungler, 1991).

OTHER TYPES OF RESEARCH

Additional types of research are discussed in this section. These types of research include: case studies, evaluation research, field studies, historical research, needs assessments, pilot studies, secondary analysis, and survey research.

Case Studies

Case study research is an intensive study of the background, current status, or environmental interactions of an individual, group, institution, or community (Isaac & Michael, 1987). Such studies may or may not be viewed as experimental, depending on how the case study is conducted (Shearer, 1982). Most case studies are nonexperimental, descriptive studies which examine relationships among different variables or trends over time (Polit & Hungler, 1991). Some case studies, however, are experimental and referred to as single subject experiments. Single subject designs are discussed further in Chapter 5. Case study approaches are also referred to as idiographic single-system designs, intrasubject designs, experimental case study designs, one-subject studies, and small-N designs (Ottenbacher, 1990; Shearer, 1982).

The primary strength of case study research is that it sometimes is the only method available for studying some phenomena when few subjects are available or when financial restrictions preclude the use of other types of study (Ventry & Schiavetti, 1986). Moreover, case studies provide information about individual subjects that is often lost in experimental designs (Weiner & Eisen, 1985). In some instances, case studies should be considered pilot studies because they need to be combined with appropriate follow-up studies using larger numbers of subjects having the same phenomena and focusing on specific hypotheses (Isaac & Michael, 1987). Table 4–3 presents several case studies that have been done in communication disorders.

On the other hand, case studies also have weaknesses. Because of their narrow focus on a few subjects, case studies are limited in their generalizability. Also, case studies are vulnerable to subjective bias. This may happen because the subject was selected because of dramatic or typical attributes. Objectivity also may be a problem because "the case . . . neatly fits the researchers preconceptions" (Isaac & Michael, 1987, p. 48).

Evaluation Research

Evaluation research involves collection and analysis of information related to the effects of a program, policy, or procedure (Hegde, 1994; Polit & Hungler, 1991). Four types of evaluation research have been described in the literature: process or implementation evaluation, outcome and impact evaluation, cost-benefit analysis, and comprehensive evaluation. This type of research can be used to assure compliance with ESB (ASHA, 1992) and PSB (ASHA, 1990a) standards for program self-analysis. It can also be used to determine treatment efficacy (Ellrodt, 1993; Frattali, 1990, 1991; Micheli, 1992; Olswang, 1990; Theil, 1992).

Process Evaluation

Process or implementation evaluation is designed to answer questions about the function of a program or policy (Polit & Hungler, 1991). Typically, this type of research involves intensive examination of a program and often involves collection of both qualitative and quantitative data gathered through interviews with clients and staff, observation of the program in operation, and analysis of records related to the program.

A process or implementation evaluation may focus on improving a new or ongoing program. Such an evaluation is sometimes referred

TABLE 4–3. Examples of Case Studies in Communication Disorders

Author(s)	Topic
Bedrosian and Willis (1987)	Effects of treatment on the topic performance of a school age child.
Collins and associates (1993)	Severe paradoxical dysphonia in two women.
Damico (1988)	Lack of efficacy in language therapy.
Dyson and Lombardino (1989)	Phonologic ability of a preschool child with Prader-Willi syndrome.
Edmonston (1982)	Speech-language management for a child with Prader-Willi syndrome.
Guitar, Kopff Schaefer, Donahue-Kilburg, and Bond (1992)	Parent verbal interaction and speech rate in stuttering.
Hargrove (1982)	Misarticulated vowels.
Hartman, Daily, and Morin (1989)	Superior laryngeal nerve paresis and psychogenic dysphonia.

(continued)

TABLE 4–3. *(continued)*

Author(s)	Topic
Harrison, Silman, and Silverman (1989)	Contralateral acoustic-reflex growth function in a client with a cerebellar tumor.
Mahr and Leith (1992)	Psychogenic stuttering of adult onset.
Miller, Miller, and Madison (1980)	Speech-language clinician's involvement in a PL 94-142 public hearing.
Monahan (1986)	Treatment of phonological processes.
Pecyna (1988)	Rebus symbol communication training.
Pollock and Schwartz (1988)	Structural aspects of phonological development.
Proctor (1990)	Oral language comprehension using hearing and tactile aids.
Schlip (1986)	Use of cued speech to correct misarticulation of /s/ and /z/.

Wing (1990)

Defective infant formulas and expressive language problems.

Windsor, Doyle, and Seigel (1994)

Language acquisition after mutism.

to as a formative evaluation. In other instances, the evaluation may be designed primarily so that the program can be replicated by others (Polit & Hungler, 1991).

Outcome and Impact Evaluation

Outcome and impact evaluation is concerned with the effectiveness of a program. In other words, its purpose is to determine whether a program should be discontinued, replaced, modified, continued or replicated. The evaluation may be referred to as a summative evaluation. An outcome evaluation is fairly descriptive but does not utilize a vigorous experimental design (Polit & Hungler, 1991). Such an evaluation documents the extent to which the goals of the program are achieved and the extent to which positive outcomes result.

Impact evaluation is designed to identify the impact(s) of an intervention, in other words, the impact(s) that can be attributed to the intervention rather than to other factors. Polit and Hungler (1991) believe that impact evaluation usually involves "an experimental or quasi-experimental design, because the aim of such evaluations is to attribute a casual influence to the specific intervention" (p. 200). Hegde (1994) agrees to an extent because he feels that "in some ways, an impact evaluation resembles experimental research. However, in practice, appropriate experimental methods are not used in impact evaluation" (p. 101).

Cost-benefit Analysis

Evaluations that determine whether the benefits of the program outweigh the cost are referred to as cost-benefit analyses. Such analyses are often done in conjunction with impact evaluations (Polit & Hungler, 1991).

Comprehensive Evaluation

Evaluation research combines process and outcome-impact evaluations which were previously described. Hegde (1994) believes that comprehensive evaluation is the only truly useful type of evaluation research because the usefulness of only process or impact evaluation is limited. A comprehensive model of evaluation which includes multiple types of evaluation was described by Isaac and Michael (1987) and is presented in Figure 4–2. The greatest problem with evaluation research is

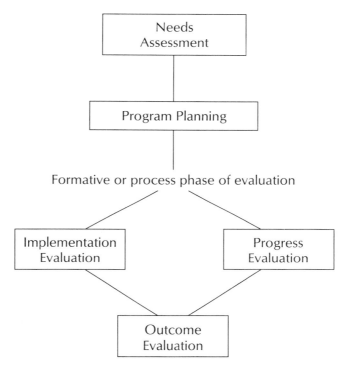

Figure 4–2. Comprehensive Model of Evaluation from Needs Assessment to Outcome Evaluation. (Adapted from *Handbook in research and evaluation* by S. Isaac and W. B. Michael, 1987, p. 5. San Diego, CA: Edits Publishers.)

that it can be threatening to individuals. Even though the focus of evaluation research is on a program, procedure, or policy, people develop and implement the entity. Sometimes people think they or their work are being evaluated. It can also be difficult to determine goals of the program (Polit & Hungler, 1991). Often the objectives of a program are multiple and diffuse.

Field Studies

Field studies are in-depth studies of individuals or groups of people conducted in naturalistic settings, that is, the "field." Field research is sometimes referred to as case research (Isaac & Michaels, 1987). It usually involves the analysis of qualitative data collected through observation, conversations with subjects, and examination of available documents (Polit & Hungler, 1991). Usually the primary difficulty with field studies is obtaining access into the group being studied.

Historical Research

Historical research, sometimes referred to as archival or library research, is a type of research aimed at establishing facts and relationships about past events (Bordens & Abbott, 1988; Polit & Hungler, 1991; Shearer, 1982). It may summarize a specific topic, sometimes in a type of review article entitled "State of the Art" or "Tutorial." Tutorial papers have been published about a variety of topics in communication disorders: facilitated communication (Duchan, 1993); hearing loss, speech, and hearing aids (Van Tasell, 1993), nonlinear-phonology (Bernhardt & Stoel-Gammon, 1994); prevention of communication disorders (ASHA, 1991e), and supplementing tests of statistical significance (Young, 1993). Such papers are often written at the request of a journal editor who wants to present a summary from the viewpoint of a recognized scholar (Shearer, 1982).

Shearer (1982) pointed out that "nearly every example of published research contains a miniature library study as part of the introductory section which refers to related research. More extensive reviews of the literature commonly comprise the second chapter of theses and dissertations" (p. 17).

The following characteristics of historical research were identified by Isaac and Michael (1987):

1. Historical research depends on data observed by others rather than by the investigator.
2. Historical research must be rigorous, systematic, and exhaustive. Much "research" claiming to be historical is an undisciplined collection of inappropriate, unreliable, or biased information.
3. Historical research depends on two kinds of data: primary sources where the author was a direct observer of the recorded event, and secondary sources where the author reports the observation of others and is one or more times removed from the original event.
4. Two basic forms of criticism weight the value of the data: external criticism which asks "Is the document or relic authentic?" and internal criticism which asks "If authentic, are the data accurate and relevant?" This critical evaluation of the data is what makes true historical research so vigorous—in many

ways, more demanding than experimental methods (p. 45). It should be noted that the terms criticism and evidence are often used interchangeably (Leedy, 1989).

Needs Assessment

A needs assessment is similar to evaluation research because it represents an effort to provide planners or decision makers with information for action (Isaac & Michael, 1987; Polit & Hungler, 1991). It is a study in which data are collected for estimating the needs of a group, community, or organization for certain types of services or policies. Needs assessments often are undertaken as a first step in comprehensive evaluations (see Figure 4–2). ASHA's (1992e, 1992f) proposed long-range plan for 1994–1999 illustrates the use of a needs assessment to identify critical issues and develop recommendations for action. Several approaches to assessing needs are available and may be combined in a single study: key information approach, survey approach, and indicators approach. In the key information approach, information is collected about the needs of a group from key individuals who are assumed to be in a position to know those needs. A survey approach relies on data collected from a sample of the target group whose needs are being assessed. An indicators approach is based on inferences made from statistics available in existing reports or records. Regardless of the method used, the final phase of a needs assessment usually involves the development of recommendations for action which are prioritized (Polit & Hungler, 1991).

Pilot Studies

Sometimes referred to as exploratory research or preliminary study, pilot studies are designed to show that certain phenomena exist and can be identified (Shearer, 1982). They usually involve a topic for which there is little or no background information. The greatest advantage of pilot studies is that they may call attention to the importance of research possibilities in an area that has been previously ignored, thus pointing the way toward future research. Pilot studies also can save time and money on a research project that will yield nothing because a pilot study almost always provides enough data to make a decision about the advisability of further study (Isaac & Michael, 1987). There are, however, limitations of pilot studies which should be considered: the investigative method will be tried in uncertain circumstances, providing little assurance that the method will work or that it will really measure what the researcher is trying to study.

Secondary Analysis

Secondary analysis involves research that uses previously gathered data (Polit & Hungler, 1991). It may involve examining unanalyzed variables, testing unexplored relationships, focusing on a specific subsample, or changing the unit of analysis. Because secondary analysis uses existing data it has the advantage of reducing time and cost. It has the disadvantage of little or no control over data collection (Hearst & Hulley, 1988). There is also the possibility the data are inaccurate.

Meta-analysis

Meta-analysis is similar to secondary analysis because it also uses previously gathered data. In meta-analysis, statistical techniques are used to compare results across previous studies (Bordens & Abbott, 1988; Cooper, 1993). This approach has existed since the turn of the century although its use was limited until the past 20 years.

Meta-analysis provides a method for integrating and synthesizing research studies and theory development. It involves: (1) identification of relevant variables, (2) location of relevant research to review, and (3) conducting the meta-analysis (i.e., comparing or combining results across studies) (Bordens & Abbott, 1988). Cooper (1993) identified several problems in meta-analysis including publication bias, missing information, reliability, independent effect sizes, correlated moderators, and interpreting effect sizes.

Survey Research

Survey research, which is often called sample survey, is designed to provide a detailed inspection of the prevalence of conditions, practices, or attitudes in a given environment by asking people about them rather than observing them directly. Surveys can be classified by the method data are obtained: controlled observation, mail questionnaire, panel, personal interview questionnaires, and telephone interviews (Kerlinger, 1973). The most powerful type of survey data is collected through personal interview (Polit & Hungler, 1991). This method has the advantage of encouraging subject cooperation, which results in higher response rates and a better quality of data (Polit & Hungler, 1991). See Table 4–4 for these and additional advantages. Personal interviews, however, have limitations: they are rather costly and considerable time is required to conduct the interviews. A variety of formats is used for questionnaires: fill in the blank, multiple choice, true/false, and selecting a number to indicate strength of agreement or disagreement with a specific item (Johnson, 1991).

The most common and easiest way to distribute questionnaires is through the mail (Bordens & Abbott, 1988). According to Shearer (1982), "surveys conducted by mail are only as effective as the form provided for the subjects' response, and a one-or-more page checklist stands a much better chance of return than does a five page list of complicated items" (p. 12). Advantages of questionnaires are listed in Table 4–4. This method has the disadvantage of nonresponse bias, (i.e., low response rates). High response rates are important for at least three reasons: (1) they increase sample size and statistical power, (2) they tend to produce a more representative sample, and (3) they reduce wasted time and materials (Dodd, Boswell, & Litwin, 1988). A response rate of 50% is considered adequate, a response rate of at least 60% is good, and a response rate of 70% or more is very good (Babbie, 1973). Questionnaires also have the disadvantage of potential bias because not all questionnaires are returned, and the ones that are returned may not be an unbiased representation of the population (Ventry & Schiavetti, 1986). Shewan (1986) suggests pretesting questionnaires so that potential problems can be identified prior to the actual mailing. Answers to the following questions are requested:

1. How long did it take you to complete the questionnaire?
2. Did you understand the instructions? What, if anything, was unclear?
3. Did you ever feel forced to make a choice that didn't fit your particular situation? If so, on which question(s) and why?
4. Were the questions reasonable and appropriate? How, in your judgment, could the questions be improved?

Polit and Hungler (1991) and Woodward (1988) also recommend pretesting of questionnaires. A cover letter should accompany mailed questionnaires, briefly explaining the purpose of the survey, conveying the researcher's thanks and appreciation for the reply, and offering to provide a summary of the results on request. A self-addressed envelope should be enclosed for returning the completed questionnaire (Shearer, 1982). Several comprehensive texts about surveys are available (Babbie, 1973; Biemer et al., 1991; Dillman, 1978; Groves, 1989; Groves et al., 1989).

TABLE 4–4. Comparison of Personal Interviews and Questionnaires

Advantages of **Personal Interviews**		Advantages of **Questionnaires**	
Clarity:	Clarify questions; avoid problem of illiteracy.	*Economy:*	Self-administration reduces staff time.
Complexity:	Obtain more complex answers and observations about respondent's appearance and behavior.	*Standardization:*	Written instructions reduce biases from differences in administration or from interactions with interviewer.
Completeness:	Minimize omissions and inappropriate responses.	*Anonymity:*	Privacy encourages candid, honest answers to sensitive questions.
Control:	Order sequence of questions.		

Source: From Planning the Measurements, in questionnaire by S. R. Cummings, W. Strull, M. C. Nevitt, and S. B. Hulley. In S. P. Hulley, and S. R. Cummings (Eds.), 1988, *Designing Clinical Research,* p. 43, Baltimore: Williams & Wilkins, with permission. Copyright 1988 Williams & Wilkins.

Questionnaires have been used to study a variety of topics in speech-language pathology and audiology (see Table 4–5). The American Speech-Language-Hearing Association routinely uses questionnaires to study such things as salaries or personal and professional characteristics of its members and reports these findings periodically in *Asha*. ASHA also conducts an annual Omnibus Survey to obtain information about professional issues of interest and concern to its members and affiliates. For example, Keough (1990) reported on results of the 1990 Omnibus Survey concerning issues such as employment and earnings and professional and continuing education. The 1991 Omnibus Survey (ASHA, 1991d) included data about equipment and supplies, caseloads, support personnel, and members' political views. In the 1992 Omnibus Survey, Slater (1992) provided data about a professional or clinical doctorate, child care, and gender issues such as discrimination and mentoring. Questionnaires also have been used to assess client satisfaction as a measure of the quality of speech-language-hearing services (ASHA, 1989a; Girolametto, Tannock, & Siegal, 1993; Rao, Goldsmith, Wilkenson, & Hildebrandt, 1992; Shipley & McCroskey, 1978).

Strengths and Weaknesses of Survey Research

The use of surveys makes it possible to obtain a great deal of information from a large population (Kerlinger, 1973). They are also economical because of the amount and quality of information they yield. Surveys, however, have a number of weaknesses. First, survey research tends to be relatively superficial; in other words, it does not usually penetrate much below the surface (Kerlinger, 1973; Polit & Hungler, 1991). Second, like ex post facto research, survey research does not permit cause-and-effect conclusions because of a lack of experimental manipulation (Hegde, 1994; Kerlinger, 1973; Polit & Hungler, 1991). A third weakness is that surveys tend to be demanding of time and other resources (Kerlinger, 1973; Polit & Hungler, 1991). Another weakness is that survey research tends to focus on soft dependent variables (Hegde, 1994).

SUMMARY

This chapter has provided an overview of the different types of research. The types of research were grouped into four categories: experimental, quasi-experimental, nonexperimental, and other types of research. Nonexperimental research includes descriptive and ex post facto

TABLE 4–5. Survey Research Published in ASHA Journals Between 1990 and 1994

Author(s)	Topic	Method of Data Collection
Allen, Pettit, and Sherblom (1991)	Management of vocal nodules	Questionnaire (mail)
Baxley and Bowers (1992)	Supervisors and supervisees' perceptions of clinical report writing	Questionnaire
Bebout and Arthur (1992)	Cross-cultural attitudes toward speech disorders	Questionnaire
Blood (1994)	Communication needs of patients after laryngectomy	Survey
Chermak and Wagner-Bitz (1993)	Speech-language pathologists' and audiologists' knowledge of clinical genetics	Questionnaire
Cooper, Bernthal, and Creaghead (1991)	Council of graduate programs	Survey
Coren and Hakstian (1992)	Pure tone threshold hearing sensitivity	Questionnaire
Coufal, Steckelberg, and Vasa (1991)	Training and utilization of paraprofessionals	Questionnaire (mail)

Author	Topic	Method
Dunn, van Kleeck, and Rossetti (1993)	Roles and needs of speech-language pathologists working in neonatal intensive care units	Telephone; Questionnaire
Fimian, Lieberman, and Fastenau (1991)	Occupational stress in speech-language pathologists	Questionnaire
Flannagin and Newman (1991)	Clinic coordinators in ESB programs	Questionnaire (mail)
Girolametto, Tannock, and Siegel (1993)	Consumer evaluation of language intervention	Questionnaire
Halls, Larrigan, and Madison (1991)	Comparison of rural and urban speech-language pathologists	Questionnaire (mail)
Henri (1994)	Graduate student preparation	Questionnaire (mail)
Hux, Morris-Friche, and Sanger (1993)	Language sampling practices	Questionnaire
Johnson, Stein, and Lass (1992)	Public school nurses' training for hearing aid monitoring	Questionnaire

(continued)

TABLE 4–5. (continued)

Author(s)	Topic	Method of Data Collection
Lass and associates (1990)	College students' knowledge and awareness of hearing, hearing loss, and hearing health	Questionnaire
Lass, Woodford, and Everly-Myers (1992)	Teachers' perceptions of stutterers	Questionnaire
Lass and associates (1993)	Speech-language pathologists career development and satisfaction	Questionnaire
Malinoff and Spivak (1991)	Professional doctorate	Questionnaire (mail)
McHalffey and Pannbacker (1992)	Stress in speech-language pathology students	Questionnaire
Morrow and associates (1993)	Vocabulary selection for augmentative communication systems	Questionnaire
Neeley, McDaniel, and Perez (1991)	NSSLHA	Questionnaire (mail)

Pannbacker, Lass, and Middleton (1993)	Ethics education	Questionnaire (mail)
Paynter, Jordan, and Finch (1990)	Patient compliance with cleft palate team recommendations	Telephone
Pezzei and Oratio (1991)	Job satisfaction of public school speech-language pathologists	Questionnaire (mail)
Plakke (1991)	Hearing conservation training of industrial technology teachers	Questionnaire
Records, Tomblin, and Freesa (1992)	Quality of life of young adults with histories of specific language impairment	Questionnaire
Rockwood and Madison (1993)	Program selection and expectations of graduate students	Questionnaire
Ruscello and associates (1990)	Speech-language pathologists' perceptions of stutterers	Questionnaire
Ruscello and associates (1991)	Professors' perceptions of stutterers	Questionnaire

(continued)

TABLE 4–5. *(continued)*

Author(s)	Topic	Method of Data Collection
St. Louis and Durrenberger (1993)	Clinician preferences for managing disorders	Questionnaire (mail)
Stouffer and Tyler (1990)	Patient response to tinnitus	Questionnaire
Vafadar and Utt (1993)	Speech-language pathologists: social dialects	Survey – telephone
Welsh and Slater (1993)	Infant hearing impairment programs	Questionnaire
Wilson and associates (1991)	Language assessment in public schools	Questionnaire (mail)
Wolery and associates (1994)	Speech-language pathologists in preschool programs	Questionnaire (mail)
Yairi and Carrico (1992)	Pediatricians' practices and attitudes about early childhood stuttering	Questionnaire (mail)

research. The last category includes case studies, evaluation research, field studies, historical research, needs assessment, pilot studies, secondary analysis, and survey research. Differences as well as similarities among the various types of research were discussed. Examples of the types of research published in the speech-language pathology and audiology literature were presented. Also mentioned was the appropriateness of certain strategies for quality management and ASHA's standards for program self-analysis.

STUDY EXERCISES

1. Review the types of research by reading examples of each.

    a. Find two research partners. Each of you locate five of the articles listed in Table 4–1. Review the articles you found and then exchange them with your partners until you have read all 15.

    b. Locate and read one of the survey studies listed in Table 4–4.

2. What is the defining characteristic of descriptive research?

3. How may experimental studies use the results of descriptive or nonexperimental research?

4. Distinguish between an experimental study and a quasi-experimental study.

5. Recall the topic you selected in Exercise 4, Chapter 1. Give an example of a subject on your topic about which very little is known and which might be appropriately investigated by means of a descriptive study.

6. Write a preliminary plan for the descriptive study in Exercise 5 above.

7. Give an example of a subject on your topic about which a great deal is known and which might be appropriately investigated by means of an experimental study.

8. Write a preliminary plan for the experimental study in Exercise 7 above.

SUGGESTED READINGS

Babbie, E. R. (1973). *Survey research methods.* Belmont, CA: Wadsworth.

Bordens, K. S., & Abbott, B. B. (1988). *Research designs and methods.* Mountain View, CA: Mayfield. Chapter 6, Using non-experimental and quasi-experimental designs, pp. 143–168. Chapter 7, Survey research, pp. 169–196. Meta-analysis, pp. 519–529.

Bradburn, N. M., & Sudman, S. (1991). The current status of questionnaire design. In P. O. Biemen, R. M. Groves, L. E. Lyboug, N. A. Mathiowetz, & S. Sudna, (Eds.), *Measurement errors in surveys* (pp. 29–40). New York: John Wiley.

Campbell, D. T., & Stanley, J. C. (1963). *Experimental and quasi-experimental designs for research.* Chicago: Rand McNally College Publishing Company.

Cummings, S. R., Strull, W., Nevitt, M. C., & Hulley, S. B. (1988). Planning the measurements: Questionnaires. In S. B. Hulley & S. R. Cummings (Eds.), *Designing clinical research* (pp. 42–52). Baltimore: Williams & Wilkins.

Hearst, N., & Hulley, S. P. (1988). Using secondary data. In S. B. Hulley & S. R. Cummings (Eds.), *Designing clinical research* (pp. 53–62). Baltimore: Williams & Wilkins.

Hegde, M. N. (1994). *Clinical research in communicative disorders.* Austin, TX: Pro-Ed. Chapter 4, Types of research, pp. 77–106.

Huck, S. W., Cormier, W. H., & Bounds, W. G. (1974). *Reading statistics and research.* New York: HarperCollins. Chapter 11, Pseudo-experimental designs, pp. 226–241. Chapter 12, True experimental designs, pp. 243–267. Chapter 13, Extensions of the basic time experimental designs, pp. 270–299. Chapter 14, Quasi-experimental designs, pp. 301–329.

Isaac, S., & Michael, W. B. (1987). *Handbook in research and evaluation.* San Diego: Edits Publishers.

Kerlinger, F. N. (1973). *Foundations of behavioral research.* New York: Holt, Rinehart & Winston.

Leedy, P. D. (1989). *Practical research.* New York: Macmillan. Methodologies of research design, pp. 125–234.

CHAPTER 5

RESEARCH STRATEGY AND DESIGN

ANN S. OWEN, WILLIS L. OWEN, MARY H. PANNBACKER, AND GRACE F. MIDDLETON

- Research Doublespeak: Strategy versus Design
- Characteristics of Good Design
- Group Designs
- Single Subject Designs
- Summary
- Study Exercises
- Suggested Readings

All types of research have a strategy or design which permits statistical analysis of differences between and within groups of subjects (Doehring, 1988; Hegde, 1994). Several types of research were described in Chapter 4. Research strategy and design refer to the plans for answering research questions and testing research hypotheses. Some authorities differentiate between these terms; others do not. The strategy or design of a study indicates the methods and procedures used in the investigation. There are essentially two types of research designs: group designs and single subject designs. Group designs include between-subject designs, within-subject designs, and mixed group designs. There are two types of single subject designs: case studies and within-subject experimental studies. Group research designs and single subject designs are compared in Table 5–1. This chapter provides information about strategy versus design and various types of design.

RESEARCH DOUBLESPEAK: STRATEGY VERSUS DESIGN

Research has more than its share of doublespeak or confusing terminology (Lutz, 1989). Doehring (1988), in his book *Research Strategies in Human Communication Disorders,* indicated "the terminology can be confusing" (p. 34). Hegde (1994) agrees and believes terms used in the description of research designs are sometimes confusing. The distinction between research strategy and research design itself is confusing. Kerlinger (1973) defines *research design* as "the plan, structure, and strategy of investigation" (p. 300). Strategy is more specific than design. On the other hand, Bordens and Abbott (1988) use strategy to imply the general plan of an investigation, and design more specifically as a procedure used to carry out the strategy. Others use the term design to refer to the overall plan of an investigation (Hegde, 1994; Polit & Hungler, 1991). Silverman (1993) uses design as a general term to refer both to overall and specific aspects of an investigation. For example, he refers to ex post facto and retrospective designs as well as single subject and group designs. Hegde (1994) combines the terms and refers to group design strategy.

CHARACTERISTICS OF GOOD DESIGN

Good research design may be described in terms of a number of characteristics. The first characteristic is the control of extraneous variables that have an irrelevant association with the dependent variable but could influence the results of the study. Essentially, there are two types of

TABLE 5–1. Comparison of Group and Single Subject Designs

Group Designs	Single-Subject Designs
Compare at least 2 groups from a target population.	Compare within subject performance for 1 subject or a small group of subjects.
Minimum number of subjects: 10	Minimum number of subjects: 1.
Outcome measures collected infrequently; usually only pre- and posttest.	Performance repeatedly measured over a period corresponding to requirements of design.
Unnecessary to run subjects more than once under each experimental condition.	Necessary to run subject more than once under each experimental condition.
Little or no subject feedback; emphasis on outcome.	Subject feedback monitored; emphasis on both process and outcome.
Inflexible; changes not permitted once intervention is introduced.	Flexible, permits addition or elimination.
Standardized measurement procedures and comparisons between subjects.	Measurement procedures flexible, individualized.

(continued)

105

TABLE 5-1. *(continued)*

Group Designs	Single-Subject Designs
Generalizable.	Not generalizable.
Expensive.	Inexpensive.
Statistical procedures well developed.	Statistical procedures relatively new.
Relatively easy to control for order and sequence effects.	Difficult to control for order and sequence effects.

Sources: "Clinically Relevant Designs for Rehabilitation Research: The Idiographic Model" by K. J. Ottenbacher, 1990, *American Journal of Physical Medicine and Rehabilitation, 69,* 286–292; *Research Design and Evaluation in Speech-Language Pathology and Audiology* by F. H. Silverman, 1993, Englewood Cliffs, NJ: Prentice-Hall; and "Group Designs in Clinical Research by G. M. Siegel and M. A. Young, 1987, *Journal of Speech and Hearing Disorders, 52*(3), 194–199.

extraneous variables: (1) intrinsic and (2) extrinsic (Polit & Hungler, 1991). *Intrinsic variables* are variables associated with subjects of an investigation such as age, gender, socioeconomic status, and marital status. There are a number of ways of reducing intrinsic variability such as randomization, homogeneity, blocking, matching, analysis of covariance, and repeated measures. *Extrinsic variables* are variables associated with the research situation or environment. These variables are related to the place and time the research was conducted and adherence or nonadherence to the research specifications or protocols. The most effective method of controlling external factors relates to the consistency of conditions under which an investigation is performed, that is, the conditions under which data are collected should be as similar as possible for every subject.

The second characteristic of good research design is that it should be appropriate for the question(s) being asked. Third, the design should result in data that are not biased. A fourth characteristic of good research is precision. Research designs differ considerably in the sensitivity with which statistically significant results can be detected. A fifth characteristic is the power of the design or its ability to detect relationships among variables. The appropriateness of research designs must also be considered relative to the current state of the art. Research designs that are today appropriate may not be appropriate in the future (Doehring, 1988).

GROUP DESIGNS

Group designs permit comparison of the average or typical performance of a group to other groups or other conditions (Warren, 1986). Several terms are used for this design: between-groups design, between-subjects design, correlational design, pre-experimental design, quasi-experimental design, and true experimental design (Bordens & Abbott, 1988; Hegde, 1994; Huck, Cormier, & Bounds, 1974).

Group designs require the formation of two or more groups for the purposes of experimentation. Groups may be formed either on the basis of matching subjects with similar characteristics or by random selection of subjects from a defined population. Hegde (1994) indicates the basic method for implementing group designs is to initially have two or more comparable groups that represent the populations from which they were drawn (especially when the random procedure is used); at least one of the groups receives a treatment variable; another group does not. Silverman (1993) describes a group design as reliably permitting the average "performance of the subjects in a group under the experimental condition or conditions to be determined" (p. 77).

Advantages and Disadvantages of Group Designs

Advantages and disadvantages of group designs are summarized in Table 5–2, and discussed briefly here. Group designs have several advantages. Statistical procedures for determining reliability are available for group designs. Another advantage is that it is possible to control order or sequence effects because relatively large numbers of subjects permit randomization (Silverman, 1993; Warren, 1986). Group designs also allow generalization of results from samples of subjects to the population as a whole (Doehring, 1988; Warren, 1986). Another advantage is the ability to demonstrate causal relationships (Doehring, 1988).

Despite the advantages of group designs, there are several disadvantages. First, is the assumption of homogeneity of group members, that is, that all members of a group respond similarly to an experimental condition. Related to this is subject attrition which can affect results because loss of group members may disrupt group equivalency (Warren, 1986). A second disadvantage is related to availability of subjects; in group designs more subjects may be required than are available (Doehring, 1988; Silverman, 1993). Third, the typical subject may not be typical, in other words, the mean or average of the group may not accurately reflect differences in individual performance (Doehring, 1988; Silverman, 1993; Warren, 1986). Fourth, it may be difficult to generalize results because of the possibility of uncertain validity (Silverman, 1993). Another disadvantage is related to limitations of quantitative information (Doehring, 1988). Last, there are ethical considerations about group designs because of concern about withholding treatment for research purposes (Warren, 1986).

Types of Group Designs

There are three types of group designs: between-subject designs, within-subject designs, and mixed subject designs. Other classifications also have been used such as simple and complex group designs (Doehring, 1988) and designs for detecting differences and designs for detecting relationships (Silverman, 1993).

Between-Subject Designs

Between-subject designs use at least two groups of subjects, each group assigned to a different level of the independent variable (Warren, 1986). An example of a between-subjects design is the study by Dromi,

TABLE 5–2. Advantages and Disadvantages of Group Designs

Advantages	Disadvantages
Reliability of data	Assumption of homogeneity of group members
Availability of statistical procedures	
	Subject attrition
Generalization from sample to population	Availability of subjects
	Typical subject may not be typical
Established population characteristics	
	Generalizability of results
Control order or sequence effects	Quantitative information
	Ethical considerations

Sources: Research Strategies in Human Communication Disorders by D. G. Doehring, 1988, Boston: College Hill Press; *Research Design and Evaluation in Speech-Language Pathology and Audiology* by F. H. Silverman, 1993, Englewood Cliffs, NJ: Prentice-Hall; and "Research Design: Considerations for the Clinician" by R. L. Warren, 1986, In R. Chapey (Ed.), *Language Intervention Strategies in Adult Aphasia* (pp. 66–80). Baltimore: Williams & Wilkins.

Leonard, and Shleiman (1993) on the grammatical morphology of Hebrew-speaking children with specific language impairment. In these designs, each treatment (combination of levels of the independent variables) is administered to separate groups of subjects. There are three classifications of between-subject designs: (1) two groups or multiple groups; (2) single factor or multifactor, and (3) univariate or multivariate. The design is parametric if the independent variable(s) take(s) on three or more quantitative values. Other between-subjects designs are nonparametric.

Multiple control group design is a variation of the single factor, multiple group design. This design uses multiple control groups because a single control group is inadequate for assessing the impact of each potentially confounding factor of the dependent variables. Multiple control groups can be included in both parametric and nonparametric designs (Bordens & Abbott, 1988). For example, Thal and Tobias (1994) studied the relationships between language and gesture in normally developing and late-talking toddlers using multiple control groups.

Factorial designs manipulate two or more independent variables; one group in the design accounts for each possible combination of the levels of the independent variables. A factorial design has two or more independent variables which are manipulated simultaneously; it permits analysis of the main effects of the independent variables separately and the interaction effects of these variables (Polit & Hungler, 1991). This design provides maximum information at less expense because it is possible to assess the main effect of each independent variable and any interactions among the variables in one experiment (Bordens & Abbott, 1988). For example, Montgomery (1993) used a factorial design to study the effects of response modality on haptic recognition in children with specific language impairments. In another example of factorial design, Bosshardt (1993) studied short-term recall and recognition performance differences between stutterers and nonstutterers.

Multivariate designs involve two or more dependent variables, and provide information about the effect of the independent variable on each dependent variable and on a composite dependent variable formed from a weighted combination of the individual dependent variables. In a multivariate design, Gutierrez-Clellen and Heinrichs-Ramos (1993) examined the referential cohesion of the narratives of Spanish-speaking children.

The validity of between-subject experimental designs can be confounded or damaged by a variety of sources such as nonrandomization, experimenter bias, and poor planning and execution of experimental conditions. Confounding can be avoided by randomization, use of blind or double-blind techniques, and careful planning of experimental conditions and of potential alternative explanations for findings (Bordens & Abbott, 1988).

Within-Subjects Designs

In within-subjects designs every subject in the experiment is exposed to all of the experimental or treatment conditions. Fewer subjects are required for this design than for an equivalent between-subjects design. Sometimes referred to as a repeated measures design, within-subjects designs are a group of designs that incorporate the same basic structure, that is, using the same subjects in all conditions (Bordens & Abbott, 1988). Within-subjects designs are classified or described similarly to between-subject designs and include two treatment, single factor, multilevel, factorial, multiple control group, and multivariate designs.

The advantages of within-subjects designs include fewer subjects required, matching of subject factors, and power in detecting effects of dependent variables. Disadvantages include less power than equivalent between-subject designs if the dependent variable is only weakly related to subject differences, and possible carryover effects when exposure to one treatment influences behavior in a subsequent treatment. Carryover can be reduced by randomizing the order of presentation of levels of the independent variable. More frequently, counter-balancing is used in which individual subjects are exposed to the treatments in different orders. Making treatment order an independent variable makes it possible to determine whether carryover effects are present and, if so, their magnitude and direction. Despite the advantages of making treatment order an independent variable, there are disadvantages. The primary disadvantage is that every treatment order requires a separate group of subjects which must be tested under every treatment condition. This is expensive in terms of number of subjects and the time required to test them. Gerratt and associates' (1993) comparative study of internal and external standards for judgments of voice quality used a within-subjects design.

Mixed Group Designs

Mixed designs combine within-subjects and between-subjects designs and are used to investigate the effects of treatment for which carryover effects would be a problem while repeatedly sampling behavior across time or trials. Such designs are also referred to as combined designs or split plot designs. Warren (1986) considers mixed group designs both descriptive and experimental. Three advantages of mixed designs are ease of implementation, generalizability of findings, and availability of statistical techniques. Frequent misinterpretation and overinterpretation of the results are the primary disadvantages. Stager and Ludlow's (1993) study of speech production changes under fluency-evoking conditions in nonstuttering speakers is an example of a mixed research design. Another example of a mixed design is Demorest and Bernstein's (1991) study of variability in speech reading sentence.

The *nested design* is a variation of the mixed group design which combines within-subjects and between-subjects designs. It involves more than one task for each level of the independent variable. For example, assume that you were conducting an experiment on the ability to write diagnostic reports. The between-subjects factor might be difficulty (low, moderate, and high). Under each level of difficulty two sets of diagnostic data would be included, with all subjects in each level of difficulty completing both sets of reports. By demonstrating the effect of item difficulty with different tasks, effects are not limited to a specific type of problem. This design is useful when subjects must be tested in groups rather than individually. It also has the advantage of increasing the generality of results (Bordens & Abbott, 1988).

Clement and Wijner (1994), in a study of vowel contrasts, analyzed their data utilizing a "three-way ANOVA, with factors subject group, vowel, and subject (nested under subject group)" (p. 86). It is important to note that subjects are always nested under subject group. An example of a nested design, with speech-language pathologists nested within states, follows:

> A group of six speech-language pathologists, two each from Louisiana, Oklahoma, and Texas, were discussing the treatment of patients with spasmodic dysphonia. The speech-language pathologists from Louisiana decided that Botox injections were the best means of treatment; therefore, their patients were injected with Botox, received no voice management, and were re-evaluated 3 months later to determine the amount of improvement. The speech-language pathologists from Oklahoma decided that voice management coupled with Botox injections were the best means of treatment; therefore, their subjects were injected, received voice management for 3 months, and then were re-evaluated to determine the amount of improvement. The speech-language pathologists in Texas decided that voice management was the best means of treatment; therefore, their patients received voice management for 3 months and then were re-evaluated to determine amount of improvement. All data were then analyzed statistically.

Further information about nested designs may be found in Hoaglin, Mosteller, and Tukey (1991).

SINGLE SUBJECT DESIGNS

Single subject designs focus on the behavior of one or a few subjects. These designs are also referred to as applied behavioral analysis designs or behavioral analysis, idiographic designs, single subject experimental designs, single case designs, intrasubject replication designs, small N-approach, and within-subjects designs. The use of the term "within-subjects designs" is confusing because it is also used to refer to a variety of group designs (Hegde, 1994).

It is misleading to consider any design that uses one or a few subjects as a single subject design. Designs that use single subjects also can be classified as case studies or single subject designs (Warren, 1986). Single subject designs are experimental designs that attempt to establish cause-and-effect relations (Hegde, 1994). On the other hand, case studies are not experimental (see Chapter 4).

Bordens and Abbott (1988) described five characteristics of single subject designs:

1. Individual subjects are observed intensely under each of several treatment conditions; these observations provide a baseline against which any future change induced by the independent variable can be evaluated.

2. All incidental variables that may affect the dependent variable are controlled as rigidly as possible.
3. Each subject is observed under all treatment conditions, and each treatment is repeated at least twice during the course of the experiment. This repetition of intrasubject replication shows the reliability of the findings.
4. Subjects usually remain in each treatment of the experiment until the behavioral measure meets a stability criterion.
5. If more than one subject is used, the additional subjects are included to evaluate the generality of findings across subjects. This intersubject replication establishes whether the results obtained with one subject are similar or dissimilar to those obtained with other subjects. (p. 263)

One of the primary characteristics that distinguishes single subject designs from group designs is the replication of treatment effects within individual subjects (Hegde, 1994). Table 5–1 further compares single subject and group designs (Bordens & Abbott, 1988; Silverman, 1993).

There are many types of single subject designs but two basic categories of single subject designs, baseline designs and discrete trials designs, have been identified (Bordens & Abbott, 1988). *Baseline designs* include designs that manipulate a single independent variable (single factor designs), those that manipulate two or more independent variables (multifactor designs), and those that measure several dependent variables (multiple baseline designs). In baseline designs the variable(s) is measured prior to the experimental treatment of intervention. Single factor designs include a baseline condition (A) during which a baseline of subject performance is established and a treatment or intervention condition (B) in which the effect of the treatment is observed. There are several types of these designs including AB, ABA, ABAB, ABAC and BAB designs (Silverman, 1993; Weiner & Eisen, 1985). These symbols are designed as follows:

A = baseline
B = first treatment or intervention
C = second treatment or intervention different from first.

Multifactor baseline designs include more than one independent variable and require that different combinations of the independent variables be tested across the study. The effects of the independent variables and their interactions can be assessed. A factorial design may be used or specific combinations may be evaluated (Bordens & Abbott, 1988). These designs can be very time consuming because each treatment is evaluated at least twice for intrasubject replication.

Multiple baseline designs involve observation of different behaviors and establishing baselines for each. Thus several behaviors are observed within the experimental context to provide multiple baselines. Treatment is then introduced separately and staggered for each behavior over time. Treatment is considered effective if the level of each behavior changes after the treatment is applied to it. These designs are also known as multiple scheduled, multielement, alternating treatments, and simultaneous designs (Weiner & Eisen, 1985).

In single subject *discrete trials designs*, individual subjects receive each treatment condition of the experiment dozens of times. Each treatment or trial produces one data point for each dependent variable measured. Extraneous variables that could introduce unwanted variability in the dependent measure are rigidly controlled. If possible, the order of treatments is randomized or counterbalanced to control order effects. Intersubject replication is established by comparing the behavior of individual subjects undergoing the same treatments.

The advantages and disadvantages of single subject designs are summarized in Table 5–3. Single subject designs often are used to determine treatment efficacy (Connell & McReynolds, 1988; Hegde, 1994; Vetter, 1985; Weiner & Eisen, 1985). These designs are economical in

TABLE 5–3. Advantages and Disadvantages of Single Subject Designs

Advantages	Disadvantages
Control of error variance	Limited generalization
Establish causal relationships	Control of extraneous variables
Identify individual differences	Control of order and sequence effects
Flexibility	
Small number of subjects (as few as 1)	Limited availability of statistical procedures
Focus on actual behavioral outcomes	
Practical clinical application	
Economical	

Sources: Research Design and Methods by K. S. Bordens and B. B. Abbott, 1988, Mountain View, CA: Mayfield; and *Research Design and Evaluation in Speech-Language Pathology and Audiology* by F. H. Silverman, 1993, Englewood Cliffs, NJ: Prentice-Hall.

terms of time because single subject research frequently can be conducted during regular clinical hours and during regularly scheduled treatment sessions (McReynolds & Thompson, 1986). Furthermore, single subject designs are similar in form to the design of therapy and are the best, if not the only, appropriate strategy to advance clinical knowledge and to assess treatment efficiency (Siegel & Young, 1987). Table 5–4 provides examples of studies using single subject research designs published in ASHA journals between 1990 and 1994. Sixty-five single subject research designs published between 1976 and 1985 were identified by Connell and Thompson (1986).

SUMMARY

Group research designs require the formation of two or more groups. Single subject designs are based on individual subject's performance under different conditions. Although group designs are often used, they do not meet the practical needs of speech-language pathologists and audiologists to evaluate treatment. These designs were described as if they were mutually exclusive, but this is not so. Some studies use designs that generate both types of data. Different study designs have different strengths and weaknesses. It is important to remember that research designs that are appropriate today may not be in the future.

STUDY EXERCISES

1. Distinguish between strategic planning and experimental design.

2. Distinguish between group and single subject designs. What are the advantages and disadvantages of each?

3. Review the list of references for single subject studies in Table 5–4. Find one about the topic you selected in Exercise 4, Chapter 1. Read the article for a practical understanding of the single subject design.

4. Read an article that reflects the use of a group design. Which type of group design was used in the study?

SUGGESTED READINGS

Bordens, K. S., & Abbott, B. B. (1988). *Research designs and methods.* Mountain View, CA: Mayfield. Part II, Research designs, pp. 141–290.

TABLE 5–4. Examples of Single Subject Research Designs in Speech-Language Pathology and Audiology

Author(s)	Topic
Abraham (1993)	Differential treatment of phonological disability in children with impaired hearing who were trained orally.
Bourgeois (1992)	Evaluating memory wallets in conversations with persons with dementia.
Casby (1992)	Intervention approach for naming problems in children.
Elbert and associates (1990)	Generalization to conversational speech.
Gierut (1992)	Evaluation of minimal pair treatment in phonological change.
Gilliam, Roussos, and Anderson (1990)	Supervisory effectiveness.
Gow and Ingham (1992)	Effect on stuttering of changing phonation intervals.
Hambrecht and Sarris (1993)	Self-supervision training with beginning clinicians.
Hillis (1993)	Ongoing assessment in the management of stuttering.
Hoffman, Norris, and Monjure (1990)	Comparison of process targeting and whole language treatments for phonologically delayed preschool children.
Light and associates (1992)	Instructing facilitators to support the communication of people who use augmentative systems.
Mineo and Goldstein (1990)	Generalized learning of action-object responses by language-delayed preschoolers.

Powell, Elbert, and Dinnsen (1991)	Stimulability and generalization of misarticulating preschool children.
Pratt, Heintzelman, and Deming (1993)	IBM Speech Viewer vowel accuracy model for treating young children with hearing impairment.
Rice, Buhr, and Oetting (1992)	Effect of a pause on language-impaired children's learning of words.
Shriberg, Kwiatkowski, and Synder (1990)	Tabletop versus microcomputer assisted speech management.
Venn and associates (1993)	Effects of teaching preschool peers to use mand-model procedure during snack activities.
Violette and Swisher (1992)	Echolalic responses by a child with autism to experimental conditions of sociolinguistic input.
Warren and associates (1993)	Facilitating prelinguistic communication skills in young children with developmental delay.
Weismer, Murray-Branch, and Miller (1993)	Comparison of two methods for promoting vocabulary in late talkers.
Williams (1991)	Generalization patterns associated with training least phonological knowledge.
Yoder and associates (1993)	Following the child's lead when teaching nouns to preschoolers with mental retardation.

Campbell, D. T., & Stanley, J. C. (1963). *Experimental and quasi-experimental designs for research.* Chicago: Rand McNally College Publishing.

Connell, P. J., & Thompson, C. K. (1986). Flexibility of single subject experimental designs. Part III. Using flexibility to design or modify experiments. *Journal of Speech and Hearing Disorders, 51*(3), 214–225.

Doehring, D. G. (1988). *Research strategies in human communication disorders.* Boston: Little, Brown. Chapter 4, Basic Principles of Research Design, pp. 31–39. Chapter 5, Simple Group Research Designs, pp. 40–50. Chapter 6, Complex Group Research Designs, pp. 51–65. Chapter 7, Advantages and Disadvantages of Group Research Designs, pp. 66–71. Chapter 8, Other Research Designs, pp. 72–83.

Hegde, M. N. (1994). *Clinical research in communicative disorders.* Austin, TX: Pro-Ed. Part II, Clinical research designs, pp. 137–352.

Huck, S. W., Cormier, W. H., & Bounds, W. G. (1974). *Reading statistics and research.* New York: HarperCollins. Chapter 15, Designs for Applied Behavioral Analysis.

Kearns, K. P. (1986). Flexibility of single subject experimental designs. Part II: Design selection and arrangement of experimental phases. *Journal of Speech and Hearing Disorders, 51*(3), 204–214.

McReynolds, L. V., & Thompson, C. K. (1986). Flexibility of single subject experimental designs. Part I: Review of the basics of single-subject designs. *Journal of Speech and Hearing Disorders, 51*(3), 194–203.

Siegel, G. M., & Young, M. A. (1987). Group designs in clinical research. *Journal of Speech and Hearing Disorders, 52*(3), 194–199.

Silverman, F. H. (1993). *Research design and evaluation in speech-language pathology and audiology.* Englewood Cliffs, NJ: Prentice-Hall. Chapter 6, Single subject and group designs, pp. 75–102.

Warren, R. L. (1986). Research design: Considerations for the clinician. In R. Chapey (Ed.), *Language intervention strategies in adult aphasia* (pp. 66–79). Baltimore, MD: Williams & Wilkins.

Weiner, I. S., & Eisen, R. G. (1985, May). Clinical research: The case study and single subject designs. *Journal of Allied Health, 14,* 191–201.

C H A P T E R 6

RESEARCH PLANNING

ANN S. OWEN, WILLIS L. OWEN, AND GRACE F. MIDDLETON

- Developing Ideas for Research
- Reviewing the Literature
- Planning a Research Project
- Summary
- Study Exercises
- Suggested Readings

The essence of research is planning. In fact, no activity should be called research unless it is completely and thoroughly planned. Research planning takes place at two levels: the overall or strategic level and the specific or experimental level. Planning begins by establishing long-term goals for the research. For example, one long-term goal might be to identify the causes of stuttering and another to identify the most effective therapy for reducing stuttering. The first study might involve identifying the characteristics of various groups of stutterers and contrasting them with the characteristics of nonstutterers. The second study might involve examining the differences in the frequency of stuttering between individuals treated by various methods. These two goals cannot be achieved in a single experiment. Strategic planning, then, involves deciding on the series of experiments that need to be undertaken to achieve the desired goal(s). This involves planning a sequence of experiments or, at the very least, putting the current project into the context of previous work in the area of interest.

DEVELOPING IDEAS FOR RESEARCH

Individual experiments are designed to obtain the information needed to move forward with the strategic plan. Clearly the methods and procedures for strategic planning are different from those for designing an individual project. Planning is based on identification of gaps in the available knowledge of the subject matter based on the researcher's broad knowledge of the subject.

Research ideas come from many sources and are easy to locate if the investigator is familiar with information sources. These include published journal articles about communication disorders, study guides, and literature reviews.

Information Resources

Libraries are a major source of information and no two are alike (Horowitz, 1988). Public libraries serve the public in a variety of ways. However, most do not have the resources or the space to handle some types of research materials. The mission of academic libraries is to serve the needs of scholars, students, and researchers. Academic libraries frequently have copies of theses, dissertations, monographs, and articles available in print, online, or in CD ROM (data storage on compact disks).

Accessing the Literature

Print sources are readily available and good sources of information when a researcher is in the planning phase of a project. Print materials provide the opportunity for browsing through materials about various topics. Common print sources usually found in an academic library include *Psychological Abstracts* and *Index Medicus.* One problem with print sources is that they may be several months behind the current literature because they have to be updated, printed, and bound. Therefore, computer database searches have become popular with researchers.

The computer search technique is similar to looking manually through a reference book such as *Psychological Abstracts* or *Index Medicus* except that a computer search is much faster. Subject headings can also be combined when doing a computer search. For example, combining "spasmodic dysphonia" *and* "Botox" provides a listing of articles that contain both subjects. Combining "spasmodic dysphonia" *or* "Botox" results in a listing of articles that contain information on both subjects or each one separately. In addition to the time savings, an advantage of using computerized databases is that they are updated more frequently than print sources. Disadvantages include the fees often charged for the search and the need for the researcher to have at least minimal training prior to using a particular database.

Computer databases frequently used by researchers in communication disorders include *Conference Papers Index, Educational Resources Information Center* (ERIC), *Linguistics and Language Behavior Abstracts,* and *Science Citation Index* (SCI search) (Davis & Findley, 1990; Huth, 1990; Shearer, 1982). Additionally, several databases are the online equivalent of print sources, for example, *Medline* (*Index Medicus*), *PsycINFO* (*Psychological Abstracts*), and *CINAHL* (*Cumulative Index to Nursing and Allied Health Literature*).

CD ROM is the newest form of information retrieval and some academic libraries are acquiring databases on CD ROM. A computer specially equipped with a CD ROM drive is required to do a search and retrieve the results from these databases. CD ROM databases are updated more frequently than print sources but not as frequently as online databases. As with online databases, efficient use of CD ROM databases requires knowledge of the organization and commands used in a particular database. Some of the available CD ROM databases are *Medline, PsycLIT* (*Psychological Abstracts*), *CINAHL,* and *ERIC. PsycLIT* and *Medline* index journals that include articles about communication disorders. They index some of the same journals, but some are carried by one but not the other. Therefore, a thorough search usually involves using both (Silverman, 1993).

Computerized reference searches are relatively simple if one follows certain procedures. Before beginning a search, key words or combinations of words and phrases related to the topic should be identified (Medsen, 1992; Silverman, 1993). Huth (1990) suggests that searches be organized according to literature published within specific periods of time. He also indicates that the researcher might consider using the services of a professional searcher. Academic libraries usually have such a person available to assist researchers in determining the database that would most efficiently locate information about a particular topic (Silverman, 1993).

To do an online database search, a computer with a modem and communication software is needed. A variety of communication software is available. Some software simply allows researchers to dial into a system; they must then know how to access the database, complete the search, and download the results of the search. Other software, such as *Grateful Med,* provides assistance in preparing a search and the software executes the search and downloads the results. Usually, the more help options the software provides, the more limited the number of databases that can be searched using it. *Grateful Med,* for example, can only be used to access databases at the National Library of Medicine.

The computer search for literature is an important time saver, and investigators must become trained users of available databases. As the technology becomes less expensive, the electronic library eventually will become a reality. In the meantime, libraries with frozen or limited budgets will continue to cut journal holdings due to overwhelming increases in library costs for periodicals. It is, therefore, necessary to allocate enough time to receive some materials by interlibrary loan when reviewing available literature about a problem under investigation.

Study Guides and Literature Reviews

Compiled references also are available such as *dsh Abstracts* (1960–1984), *Dissertation Abstracts, Index Medicus, Linguistics and Language Behavior Abstracts,* and *Psychological Abstracts* (Silverman, 1993). Study guides to communication disorders review general and specific topics (Northern, 1989; Payne & Anderson, 1992). Review articles also are published periodically in speech, language, and hearing journals.

Journals Related to Communication Disorders

In addition to the six journals published by ASHA (see Table 9–2), there are more than a dozen journals devoted to communication disorders, and many more journals publish some articles related to communication disorders (Goldstein & Hockenberger, 1991; Hegde, 1994; Trudeau & Crowe, 1988). In fact, Trudeau and Crowe (1988) state that "speech-language pathologists who limit themselves to the four ASHA periodicals will be woefully lacking if only [because] they will fail to develop an interdisciplinary perspective" (p. 35). Titles of journals that include articles about topics related to communication disorders and intervention research are shown in Table 6–1. Knowledge of journals that include such articles assists the investigator in searching specific literature on topics related to communication disorders and selecting appropriate journals to submit manuscripts.

REVIEWING THE LITERATURE

The information included in the literature review is based on intensive, extensive review of available literature on a topic. The purpose of the literature review is to place research ideas in the context of the existing literature, and avoid "reinventing the wheel" (Bordens & Abbott, 1988; Findley, 1991). Reviewing the literature can prevent conducting a study that has already been done and provide guidance in designing a study. Bordens and Abbott (1988) believe that reviewing the literature can "identify variables to control, standardized tests or methods to use, types of apparatus, appropriate analytic tools" (p. 31)—just about anything needed to design a study. A major problem in searching and reviewing the literature is failing to allow enough time (Rosenblum, 1989).

Findley (1991) described a strategy to determine which articles are highly relevant to a research topic and recommended locating all relevant articles published within the past 5 years. In this strategy, articles are classified as highly relevant, less relevant, and potentially relevant. Guidelines are provided on how to begin looking for relevant articles, organize the articles so they can be reviewed in a reasonable amount of time, and review the most relevant articles in depth.

PLANNING A RESEARCH PROJECT

The spark that initiates a research project may come from almost anywhere. Frequently a project is begun because someone identifies the availability of a group of interesting subjects who may be willing to participate in a study that could fill a gap in what is known about a particular condition or disorder. Sometimes a project seems to be a

TABLE 6-1. Journals Containing Articles onTopics Related to Speech-language Pathology and Audiology*

Academy of Rehabilitative Audiology
American Annals of the Deaf
American Journal of Mental Deficiency
American Journal of Otolaryngology
American Journal of Psychiatry
Annals of Dyslexia
Annals of Otology, Rhinology, and Laryngology
Analysis of Verbal Behavior
Annual Review of Applied Linguistics
Applied Psycholinguistics
Archives of Neurology
Archives of Otolaryngology
Audecibel
Audiology and Hearing Education
Augmentative and Alternative Communication
Behavior Modification
Brain: A Journal of Neurology
Brain and Language
Child Development
Child Language Teaching and Therapy
Cognition
Cognitive Therapy and Research
Ear and Hearing
Ear, Nose and Throat Journal
Education and Training of the Mentally Retarded
European Journal of Communication Disorders
Folia Phoniatrica
Hearing Aid Journal
Hearing Instruments
International Journal of Pediatric Otorhinolaryngology
Journal of Abnormal Child Psychology
Journal of Applied Behavior Analysis
Journal of Auditory Research
Journal of Autism and Developmental Disorders
Journal of Child Language
Journal of Childhood Communication Disorders
Journal of Communication Disorders
Journal of Computer Users in Speech-Language Pathology and
    Audiology (CUSH)
Journal of Experimental Child Psychology

TABLE 6–1. *(continued)*

Journal of Fluency Disorders
Journal of Gerontology
Journal of Laryngology and Otology
Journal of Linguistics
Journal of Otolaryngology
Journal of Pediatric Otolaryngology
Journal of Psycholinguistic Research
Journal of Special Education
Journal of Special Education Technology
Journal of the Acoustical Society of America
Journal of the American Academy of Audiology
Journal of the Association for Persons with Severe Handicaps
Journal of Voice
Language Acquisition and Language Disorders
Laryngoscope
Learning and Motivation
Linguistics and Language Behavior Abstracts
Mental Retardation
Neurology
Otolaryngology: Head and Neck Surgery
Otoscope
Phonology
Psychological Review
Research in Developmental Disabilities
Rocky Mountain Journal of Communication Disorders
Seminars in Hearing
Seminars in Speech and Language
SUPERvision
Tejas
The Hearing Journal
The Cleft Palate-Craniofacial Journal
The Supervisors' Forum
Topics in Language Disorders
Volta Review

*Does not include journals published by ASHA. See Table 9–2 for ASHA publications.

logical extension of an article someone has recently read. Sometimes the project is suggested by observing that some group (of one or more subjects) has a condition or disorder that has not been observed before (e.g., Acquired Immune Deficiency Syndrome [AIDS] in 1981).

Formulating Research Questions

The most important part of clinical research is asking the right question. The way a research question is stated determines what data will be collected, how the data will be analyzed, and what conclusion or conclusions may be drawn from the study (Findley, 1989). Therefore, no matter how the initial idea originated, it is worthwhile to spend time refining and polishing the research question. The two primary principles which guide the activity of refining the research question are: (1) the question must be an important extension of the information that is already known, and (2) the question must be one which can be addressed with the resources available at this particular time.

To understand the first principle, think of a line with one end labeled 0% and the other end labeled 100%. Suppose that this line represents our knowledge about the phenomena under study. It seems clear that the questions that are appropriate if our knowledge is near zero are very different from those that are appropriate if we know a great deal about the subject. For example, in 1903 the Wright brothers were investigating whether it was possible to build an airplane. By 1953, Chuck Yeager and others were investigating ways in which it was possible to fly faster than the speed of sound. Examples of research questions that have appeared in the communication disorders literature are included in Table 6–2.

One of the most common errors made by less experienced researchers is to attempt to address research questions which will not be appropriate until some further information has been acquired. For example, in the early 1980s people began to recognize a new disease which we now call AIDS. The first studies of AIDS focused on describing the disease, determining who contracts the disease, and describing the symptoms and possible cause(s) of the disease. As knowledge of AIDS progressed, research was directed toward methods of prevention and treatment. Common errors made by students when formulating research questions are found in Table 6–3.

Stating the Problem

Identification of a problem that, if resolved, would be a valuable addition to the pool of knowledge on a topic is a critical consideration in selecting and developing a research project. The relevancy of the study to theoretical bases and/or clinical practice in speech-language pathology should also be considered. The statement of a problem is the precursor to developing a well-defined research question and design.

TABLE 6-2. Examples of Research Questions and Purpose Statements That Have Appeared in the Communication Disorders Literature

Question or Statement	Reference
Research Question	
What is the effectiveness of a voice treatment program using vocal education, abuse reduction, computer-assisted easy onset of volume and breathing information and transfer activities?	Blood (1994)
Do African American children who delete final consonants as part of a dialectical pattern systematically vary the length of vowels according to the intended final consonant?	Moran (1993)
Is it possible to modify supervisory behavior in a graduate level course?	Dowling (1993)
Does the short-term memory (STM) performance of specific language impairment (SLI) children differ from that of their language level peers?	van der Lely and Howard (1993)
Can children with developmental language disorders be divided on the basis of frequency and type of disfluencies?	Hall, Yamashita, and Aram (1993)
Purpose Statement	
The present investigation was undertaken to further examine the relationship between speech-language impairments and reading disabilities.	Catts (1993)
The aim of the present investigation was to further investigate . . . the effect of body type on respiratory kinematics during speech production to confirm, or otherwise, the existence of differences in speech breathing across subject groups comprising individuals of differing body types.	Manifold and Murdoch (1993)
This study will describe a systematic process for evaluating tests for use in identifying language impairment in preschool children.	Plante and Vance (1994)

TABLE 6-3. Common Research Errors Made by Students

Formulating a Research Study	1. Puts off selection of a problem until all or most courses are finished. 2. Uncritically accepts the first research idea thought of or suggested. 3. Selects a problem that is too vast or too vague to investigate meaningfully. 4. Prepares unclear or untestable hypotheses. 5. Fails to consider methods or analysis procedures in developing a tentative research plan.
Reviewing the Literature	1. Carries out a hurried review of the literature in order to get started. This usually results in overlooking previous studies containing ideas that would have improved the project. 2. Relies too heavily on secondary sources. 3. Concentrates on research findings when reading research articles, thus overlooking valuable information on methods, measures, etc. 4. Overlooks sources other than ASHA journals. 5. Fails to satisfactorily limit the review of the literature. 6. Copies bibliographic data incorrectly and then is unable to locate the needed reference. 7. Copies too much material on note cards.
Gathering Research Data	1. Pays insufficient attention to establishing and maintaining rapport with subjects. 2. Weakens research design by making changes for administrative convenience. 3. Fails to explain the purposes of measures used in the research to administrators. 4. Fails to evaluate available measures thoroughly before selecting those to be used. 5. Selects measures of such low reliability that true differences are hidden by the errors of the measure.

TABLE 6–3. *(continued)*

6. Selects measures not qualified to administer and score.

Standard Measuring Instruments

1. Fails to check content validity.
2. Fails to standardize or control data collection.
3. Checks overall validity and reliability of measures selected but fails to check validity and reliability data on subtest scores.
4. Uses personality inventories and other self-reporting devices in situations in which the subject might fake replies to create a desired impression.
5. Assumes that standard tests measure what they claim to measure without making a thorough evaluation of available validity data.
6. Attempts to use measures not sufficiently trained to administer, analyze, or interpret.
7. Fails to make optimum use of the testing time available.
8. Does not carry out a pretrial of measuring instruments and, as a result, makes blunders in administration procedures during the collection of first data, thus introducing bias.

Statistical Tools

1. Selects statistical tool that is not appropriate or correct for proposed analysis.
2. Collects research data, and then tries to find a statistical technique that can be used in analysis.
3. Uses only one statistical procedure when several can be applied to the data.
4. Uses statistical tools in situation in which the data grossly fail to meet the

(continued)

TABLE 6–3. *(continued)*

Statistical Tools *(continued)*	assumptions on which the tools are based. 5. Overstates the importance of small differences that are statistically significant. 6. Voids correlational analysis if the standard product-moment correlation cannot be applied. 7. Uses the incorrect correlation technique. 8. Uses the product-moment correlation significance tables to interpret non-Pearson correlations. 9. Uses correction for attenuation in situations where it is not appropriate to make the results appear more significant.
Research Design and Methodology	1. Fails to define research population. 2. Uses a sample too small to permit analysis of the performance of interesting subgroups. 3. Attempts to conduct research using volunteer subjects. 4. Changes design in ways that weaken the research to make data collection more convenient. 5. In an attempt to collect as much data as possible, makes excessive demands on subjects that lead to their refusal to cooperate. 6. Attempts to carry out a study in one semester that would require 2 or 3 years to do satisfactorily. 7. Fails to plan data collection in sufficient detail to avoid excessive treatment errors. 8. Starts collecting research data without carrying out a pilot study or adequately testing measures and procedures.
Historical Research	1. A research area is selected in which sufficient evidence is not available to conduct a worthwhile study or test the hypotheses adequately.

TABLE 6-3. *(continued)*

2. Excessive use of secondary sources.
3. Attempts to work on a broad and poorly defined problem.
4. Fails to adequately evaluate historical data.
5. Allows personal bias to influence research procedures.
6. The student's report recites facts but does not synthesize or integrate these facts into meaningful generalizations.

Descriptive Research

1. Does not formulate clear and specific objectives.
2. Relates data-gathering procedure to objectives only in a general way and thereby fails to obtain quantitative data specific to problem.
3. Selects sample on the basis of convenience rather than attempting to obtain a random sample.
4. Does not plan analysis until after data are collected.
5. Structures data collecting devices (questionnaires, interview guides, observation forms, and so on) so that biased results are obtained.

Questionnaire Studies

1. Uses a questionnaire in working with problems that can be studied better with other research techniques.
2 Gives insufficient attention to the development of questionnaire and fails to pretest it.
3. Asks too many questions, thus making unreasonable demands on the respondents' time.
4. Overlooks details of format, grammar, printing.
5. Fails to check a sample of non-responding subjects for possible bias.

(continued)

TABLE 6-3. *(continued)*

Interview Studies	1. Does not adequately plan the interview or develop a detailed interview guide.
	2. Does not conduct sufficient practice interviews to acquire needed skills.
	3. Fails to establish safeguards against interviewer bias.
	4. Does not make provisions for calculating the reliability of interview data.
	5 Uses language in the interview that is not understood by the respondents.
	6. Asks for information that the respondent cannot be expected to have.
Observational Studies	1. Does not sufficiently train observers and thus obtains unreliable data.
	2. Uses an observation form that requires too much time.
	3. Fails to take adequate safeguards against the observer disturbing or changing the situation that is being observed.
	4. Attempts to evaluate behavior that occurs so infrequently that reliable data cannot be obtained through observations.
Content Analysis	1. Selecting content that is easily available but does not represent an unbiased sample of all content related to the research objectives.
	2. Fails to determine the reliability of content-analysis procedures.
	3. Uses classification categories that are not sufficiently specific and comprehensive.
Study of Relationships	1. Assumes the results of causal-comparative or correlational research to be proof of a cause-and-effect relationship.
	2. Uses sample in causal-comparative research that differs on so many

TABLE 6–3. *(continued)*

pertinent variables that comparisons of groups can yield no interpretable results.

3. Attempts to study possible causes of a broadly defined behavior pattern that actually includes a number of unlike subgroups.

4. Tries to build a correlational study around conveniently available data instead of collecting the data needed to do a worthwhile study.

5. Selects variables for correlation that have been found unproductive in previous studies.

6. Fails to make use of theory in selecting variables for study in correlation research.

7. Uses simple correlation techniques in studies where partial correlation or multiple correlation is needed to obtain a clear picture of the way the variables are operating.

8. Applies tables giving significance levels of Pearson correlation coefficients to non-Pearson correlations, which often leads to reporting nonsignificant relationships as being significant.

9. Uses the "shotgun" approach in exploratory relationship studies.

10. Fails to develop satisfactory criterion measures for use in correlation studies of complex skills or behavior patterns.

Source: Adapted from *Educational Research: An Introduction,* by W. R. Borg, 1979, p. 38–39. New York: David McKay.

Furthermore, it is important to clearly define the problem that justifies the study. If the study is designed so that it can potentially fulfill its purpose or answer the research question, then it is assumed that the study is viable.

Making Assumptions Explicit

Prior to collecting data, the method for data analysis must be determined. There are limitations in both statistical and nonstatistical methods of analysis. Certain assumptions may be necessary to illustrate the limitations of a selected statistical or nonstatistical treatment. Also limitations of one type of analysis over another in effectively answering the question contribute to the ultimate selection of the appropriate method for analyzing the data.

For example, Catts (1993) studied the relationship between children with speech-language impairment and reading disabilities. Comparison of the reading scores of the speech-language-impaired and normal control subjects indicated a positive or definite relationship between the presence of a speech and language impairment and a reading disability. However, assuming that certain subvariables in the speech-language-impaired group more strongly affected reading than others, Catts employed a multivariate analysis of differences so that he could look at two subgroups of the speech-language-impaired sample: a language-impaired subgroup and a group with primarily articulation impairments. The language-impaired subgroup scored significantly lower on reading measures than the control group, whereas the primarily articulation-impaired group did not differ significantly from the control group on measures of reading. Some prior studies had linked reading with speech and language disorders. This study, because of the assumption that one variable in this group might be affecting reading more than another, selected a statistical treatment that could effectively identify that variable.

Measurable and Nonmeasurable Quantities

Researchers in fields such as chemistry and physics have an advantage over researchers in many other fields because the variables they study all have direct physical measurements. Researchers in fields such as communication sciences and disorders frequently want to study a variable that cannot be measured directly.

In an effort to investigate satisfaction of laryngectomees with different modes of communication, for example, the researcher is challenged by the fact that "satisfaction" is both difficult to define and cannot be measured directly. The concept of "satisfaction" must be made concrete to continue with this project. One possibility is to have each laryngectomee record and rate the intelligibility of a standard speech passage using different modes of communication. Another possibility is to have laryngectomees keep a diary to rate speech events immediately after each conversation as either "satisfactory" or "unsatisfactory." The ratings by the subjects serve to make the subjective behavior or attitude (in this case satisfaction) more concrete.

Defining the Research Population

Some researchers deal with populations that are somewhat ambiguously defined; for example, when is a difference a disorder? Also, some clinicians might classify a particular individual as having a mild disorder and other clinicians might classify the same individual as having a moderate or severe disorder. One way to solve this problem is to take a consensus of opinion of certified professionals concerning the severity of the disorder. To be precise in the definition of professionals, the researcher could state that each of them must have at least 5 current years of experience involving direct service with the disorder in question. In addition, while investigating the intelligibility of various communication devices, the researcher could set additional criteria for the judges. For example, the judges should have normal hearing and people who have listened to one type of communication device on a regular basis should be excluded from the study. In this way, the group of clinicians is precisely defined.

The population to be studied also must be defined unequivocally so that any competent professional in the field can determine whether a particular individual meets the criteria for inclusion in the study. For example, laryngectomees included in a study of the intelligibility of various communication devices could be selected based on their use of a particular communication device for at least three years and their having normal articulation skills.

Stating Specific Questions in Terms of Measurable Quantities

The design of an individual experiment begins with a clear and detailed statement of the question to be addressed by the experiment. The success of the experiment depends more on the statement of this question than on any other single factor. The paramount importance of having a well-stated question for the experiment to address becomes clear when it is realized that the entire design process consists of making plans and decisions that will permit the research question to be answered with the resources available (see Table 6–2).

The research question must be narrowed following a review of the literature and must be stated in terms of measurable quantities. New researchers often make the mistake of stating a too broad research question such as "investigating stuttering" (see Table 6–3). After reading the literature in the area, they "narrow" the topic to either the "etiology" or "treatment of stuttering". A mature researcher, on the other hand, might decide to investigate the "aerodynamic (airflow and estimated glottal pressure) of stutterers during fluent and nonfluent speech." Of course, this researcher would have to precisely define "fluent" and "nonfluent."

The research question concerns a group of subjects or a population that explicitly includes individuals in the future. The population conceptually includes individuals at some future time because researchers are interested in a therapy or preventive measures for use with persons who develop the disorder in the future. The question concerns this population even if the design is a single subject design. The technique for selecting the sample is determined so that the researcher has the best chance of obtaining a representative sample, a sample which is as like a population as possible with respect to the distribution of the variables to be measured. The population and representative sample factors must be considered in every research project, even if the design is a single subject design or if the entire project is determined by the availability of a "unique subject."

Specifying the Data Needed to Answer the Questions

After defining the population, specifying the variables to be measured, and stating the research question in measurable terms, the researcher should summarize this activity by preparing a list. The list should relate the concept being studied (e.g., voice) with the measurable quantities used to define the concept (e.g., spectral noise levels, jitter, shimmer, median roughness ratings). If the list is prepared conscientiously, it will contain all the variables that need to be collected to complete the study. Once the data have been collected, the list provides a guide to the analysis needed to answer the research question.

One pitfall of an otherwise well developed plan may be a lack of available subjects. A pilot study on a few subjects provides the researcher with valuable experience in locating subjects, collecting appropriate data, and recording it in a format readily understandable to the most likely readers or users of the research. Setting up tables, graphs, and charts and recording pilot data on them helps the researcher determine the feasibility of a research plan (Findley, 1989).

Sampling Techniques

The inferences drawn from the study cannot be better than the sample used to obtain the data. It is important to select the subjects in an objective and preplanned manner. Frequently, the sample consists of all the available subjects at a particular time and place. Such samples are treated as if they are simple random samples. A simple random sample is a sample selected in such a way that every member of the population has an equal opportunity for inclusion in the sample. Usually, when the term "random sample" is used a "simple random sample" is implied.

Bias

Some randomization technique should be used to obtain the sample. If a randomization technique is not used, there is a danger that the selection procedure may suffer from some unconscious preference of the individual doing the selecting.

The unconscious exercise of preference mentioned above is an example of bias. Simply stated, *bias* is the result of any systematic occurrence that results in a sample that in some way is not representative of the population. For example, novice researchers frequently suggest that a sample of patients be drawn from a set of clinic files by using a yardstick and selecting each file that is a whole number multiple of some set distance. A few moments of thought will persuade anyone that this selection method gives a higher probability of selecting thicker files, thus biasing the sample (see Table 6–3).

Most researchers find it necessary to expend a great deal of effort to ensure that their sample is not biased and is as representative of the population as possible. All relevant variables should be included in the study design either as study factors or as part of the criteria for entry into the study. After this has been done, it is imperative that some probability based selection technique be used to make the final subject selection or assignment.

Sampling Methods

Randomization refers to every member of the population having an equal chance of being included in the study. Randomization techniques are logically equivalent to putting names on pieces of paper and drawing them from a hat. More sophisticated randomization techniques are needed if the sample size exceeds two or three. Currently, the most common randomization techniques are to use tables of random numbers or randomization software, which is available for most computers.

CONTROLS (MATCHED). In designs that require comparison of more than one group, it is necessary to decide whether the groups will be the same size and whether some matching or pairing technique will be employed. Some researchers always use a matching technique as part of the subject selection process.

Suppose a researcher wants to study a moderately rare disorder such as spasmodic dysphonia. If two treatments are to be compared, the researcher will want the groups exposed to each treatment to be as alike as possible. Because restrictive entry into the study may severely reduce the number of subjects available, the researcher may decide to match subjects to avoid the effect of possible confounding variables. That is, a simple random division of available subjects into two groups might result in groups which are very different with respect to age. If the researcher pairs subjects according to their ages and then randomly assigns one member of each pair to each treatment group, the two groups will be alike with respect to this matching variable. Thus, the differences observed between the two groups could not be due to differences in this variable.

It should be noted that there is a controversy among statisticians concerning whether matched studies actually have advantages over unmatched studies. It is important to remember that the use of matching represents a choice made by the researcher. It is also important to remember that, if matching is used, the statistical techniques appropriate for related samples must be used.

CONTROLS (UNMATCHED). Sometimes a researcher is in the position of comparing two groups, one of which is rare and the other more abundant. In this situation it is important to include all available subjects from the rare population in the study. It is possible to improve the efficiency by selecting more subjects from the abundant group than there are subjects in the rare group. It usually is not worthwhile to have the more abundant group be more than two or three times the size of the rare group.

Power and Sample Size

Part of the design of every study should be an estimation of the power available for making the planned statistical tests and an estimation of the expected length of any confidence intervals to be calculated. *Power* is the probability of correctly rejecting a null hypothesis. It is desirable to have the probability of making a correct decision as high as possible. Furthermore, it is clearly a waste of time and money to conduct a study in which the probability of making a correct decision is low. A power analysis should be made to make sure that there are enough available subjects to make the study worthwhile.

Data Collection Forms

In almost all cases, the researcher must develop a data collection form to be used in recording the values of the variables measured. The form may be revised following a pilot study to improve the ease of data collection and prevent collection of unnecessary data (Findley, 1989). Subsequently, the form should allow easy entry of the data into a computer. The form should be developed well in advance and contain all the information that will be collected from each subject. It is preferable that this form not be crowded; it is better to use two pages than to crowd everything into one.

If some variables are to be coded when entered into the computer, the codes should be included on the form. For example, if gender will be entered into the computer as a numerical code, the code should be specified on the form (e.g., males = 1; females = 2).

The order of the items on the form should be the same order in which the items will be collected during the study. It is also helpful if the items are listed in the same order in which they will be entered into the computer.

SUMMARY

In research planning and design, it is essential that all aspects of research be defined precisely in terms of quantities that can be measured in standardized ways. Information about research topics may be accessed from a variety of sources. An intensive, extensive review of available literature is critical to the successful planning of a project. The process of formulating research questions in terms of measurable quantities, defining and locating a research population appropriate for the study, selecting appropriate sampling techniques, and specifying data needed to answer the research question are critical to a well-designed study. Additionally, data collection forms should be planned in advance of the project and should provide sufficient space to record all the necessary data.

STUDY EXERCISES

1. What are the importance and purpose of a careful search and review of the literature? How might an inadequate review of the literature affect a research project?

2. Differentiate between computerized and manual literature searches.

3. Interview an experienced researcher. During the interview, ask the following question: Have your greatest research successes resulted from following well thought out plans or from taking advantage of unanticipated opportunities (Hegde [1994] calls this serendipity)? Cite the person's answer with your comments.

4. What is the role of the research question in the design of an experiment?

5. Write a well-stated research question for the topic you selected in Exercise 4, Chapter 1.

6. How would you ensure that all subjects selected for the study of the question developed in Exercise 5 above have the same disorder and, conversely, ensure that none of the subjects would be diagnosed with a different disorder.

7. Review two research articles on the topic selected for Exercises 5 and 6 above. Review the research questions in each article. How specific and measurable are they? If you identify problems in meeting the criteria of a good research question, rewrite the question or questions so that the criteria are met.

8. Define the population you would target in the development of a study based on the question written for Exercise 5 above. Define the populations targeted in the articles you reviewed for Exercise 7 above.

9. Define the following: sample, representative sample, and bias. How would you select a random sample from each of the populations described in Exercise 8 above?

10. Assume that you are going to collect the data in each of the articles selected for Exercise 7 above. Develop a data collection form for each.

11. Make a list of 50 individuals in your program or department. Use a randomization technique to select a sample of 10 from the list. Measure the height of each of the 10 individuals and compute the average of the heights. Compare your sample with the samples obtained by the other students in your class. All samples should be selected from the same list of 50 individuals.

a. What are the highest and lowest averages?

b. How many people from the list of 50 were included in more than one sample?

c. How many people from the list of 50 were not included in any sample?

SUGGESTED READINGS

Barber, T. X. (1976). *Pitfalls in research: Ten pivotal points.* New York: Pergamon Press.

Findley, T. W. (1989). Research in physical medicine and rehabilitation. I. How to ask the question. *American Journal of Physical Medicine and Rehabilitation, 68*(1), 26–31.

Findley, T. W. (1991). Research in physical medicine and rehabilitation: II. The conceptual review of the literature or how to read more articles than you ever want to see in your entire life. *American Journal of Physical Medicine and Rehabilitation, 70*(1), 517–522.

Horowitz, L. (1988). *Knowing where to look: The ultimate guide to research.* Cincinnati, OH: Writer's Digest Books.

Rosenblum, M. (1989). Principles and practices in searching the scientific literature. In E. P. Woodford (Ed.), *Scientific writing for graduate students* (pp. 167–178). Bethesda, MD: Council of Biology Editors.

CHAPTER 7

ORGANIZATION AND ANALYSIS OF RESEARCH DATA

ANN S. OWEN, WILLIS L. OWEN, MARY H. PANNBACKER, AND GRACE F. MIDDLETON

- ■ Data Management
- ■ Qualitative Analysis
- ■ Quantitative Analysis: Descriptive Statistics
- ■ Integration of Qualitative and Quantitative Analysis
- ■ Inferential Statistics
- ■ Advanced Statistical Procedures
- ■ Summary
- ■ Study Exercises
- ■ Suggested Readings

Data must be organized and summarized after it has been collected. Several procedures for organizing and analyzing data are available including narrative description, tabular presentation, statistical analysis, and graphic display. The first two procedures are used for organizing and summarizing qualitative or non-numerical data. The last three are used for organizing quantitative or numerical data (Silverman, 1993). Speech-language pathologists and audiologists utilize these strategies more than they may realize in routine clinical practice. For example, clinicians organize and summarize qualitative data narratively in evaluation reports and daily logs of treatment sessions. The pure-tone audiogram is a graphic display for organizing quantitative data. Profile analysis involves integration of both qualitative and quantitative data (Cole, Mills, & Kelley, 1994). The availability of computers and appropriate software has revolutionized research. Computers are used throughout the research process to conduct reference searches, collect and store data, maintain administrative research records, organize and analyze data, and prepare research proposals and reports. The purpose of this chapter is to provide an overview for organization and analysis of data in speech-language pathology and audiology research.

DATA MANAGEMENT

Computers have changed the way data are collected, stored, and analyzed. The advantages of computers include speed, accuracy, and flexibility. Computers, however, require considerable attention from the user because computers are ductile or stupid; they cannot think on their own (Bordens & Abbott, 1988; Kerlinger, 1973; Polit & Hungler, 1991). The output from a computer is only as good as the user's input.

Several basic principles apply to all stages of data management (Buchner & Findley, 1990). These principles are: (1) planning for data management and analysis in advance; (2) paying attention to detail; (3) using graphs in data analysis, especially for identifying analysis problems; and (4) keeping a permanent record of what was done.

A sometimes overlooked part of research is management of the data (Feigal et al., 1988). The first stage of data management is data entry and cleaning to create a computer data file free of clerical errors (Findley & Stineman, 1989). Data is put into a form the computer can read, that is, the data are edited and prepared for entry into computer files. This includes assigning a unique identification number to each subject before entering any information into the database so the computer can identify specific clients, developing a data entry form, selecting a data entry program, and entering the data. Data are verified by visual inspection of the raw data. Statistical programs are used to locate possible errors by finding outliers, or data points that are very different (Feigal et al., 1988; Findley & Stineman, 1989). Special graphic outputs of the statistical program such as scatter plots and box and whisker plots also can be used to identify questionable data.

The second stage of data management—preliminary data analysis—is done after data are checked for clerical entry errors but before the primary statistical analysis is performed (Buchner & Findley, 1990). The purpose of preliminary data management is to prepare raw data for the primary analysis by recoding data, either to reduce data complexity or to meet the assumptions of the planned statistical tests. This involves description and graphic display of each variable, recoding categorical data, transforming continuous data into another continuous variable, and recoding continuous to categorical data. Missing values and outlying data points should be identified. Variable recording can be tedious and mistakes are common. Mistakes in recoding data can be minimized by using distinct, easy to remember variable names, noticing missing values, using graphs to check the accuracy of recoding, using variable codes consistently, and keeping a permanent record of recoding.

The third stage of data management is primary data analysis in which statistical techniques are applied to the data (Findley, 1990). Selecting the appropriate statistic depends on: (1) the number of groups: two or more than two groups; (2) relationship of the groups: composed of independent or related measures; (3) distribution of data; and (4) type of result stated in hypothesis: comparison or relationship (Shearer, 1982). Several statistical packages for computers are available (Bordens & Abbott, 1988; Feigal et al., 1988). Statistical errors are common (Colditz & Emerson, 1985). Findley (1990) identified common mistakes such as "use of standard error of the mean instead of standard deviation, use of standard deviation with skewed data, failure to describe the statistical test used, multiple comparisons and failure to use special forms of t test and X^2" (p. 209). Young (1993) pointed out that a tutorial about limitations of tests of statistical significance would be "unnecessary if authors encouraged by editors, would regularly report appropriate measures of effect size" (p. 654). Some mistakes can be avoided by using available guidelines for statistics (Aylward & Verhulst, 1991; Bailar & Mosteller, 1988; Gardner, Machin, & Campbell, 1986; McAleer, 1990; Rosenfeld, 1991; Stevens, 1991). A checklist such as that in Table 7–1 can be helpful.

The last stage of data management is secondary data analysis (Buchner & Findley, 1990). This stage uses the existing database to consider new research questions. Additional data analysis may be necessary to provide the basis for secondary analysis.

TABLE 7-1. Checklist for Assessing Research Studies

	Yes	No	Comment(s)
1. Was the objective of the study adequately described?	☐	☐	_____
2. Was an appropriate design used to achieve the objective?	☐	☐	_____
3. Was there a satisfactory statement about the source of the subjects?	☐	☐	_____
4. Was there a power based assessment of adequacy of sample size?	☐	☐	_____
5. Was the response rate satisfactory?	☐	☐	_____
6. Were all the statistical procedures used adequately referenced?	☐	☐	_____
7. Were the statistical analyses used appropriate?	☐	☐	_____
8. Was the statistical material presented?	☐	☐	_____
9. Were confidence intervals given for the main results?	☐	☐	_____
10. Were the conclusions drawn from the statistical analyses justified?	☐	☐	_____

Sources: From "Guidelines for Statistical Reporting in Articles for Medical Journals" by J. C. Bailar and F. Mosteller, 1988, *Annals of Internal Medicine, 108,* 266–273; "Research in Physical Medicine and Rehabilitation IX. Primary Data Analysis" by T. W. Findley, 1990, *American Journal of Physical Medicine and Rehabilitation, 69*(4), 209–218; and "Use of Checklists in Assessing the Statistical Content of Medical Studies" by M. J. Gardner, D. Machin, and M. J. Campbell, 1986, *British Medical Journal, 292,* 810–812.

QUALITATIVE ANALYSIS

Depending on the discipline, qualitative research is sometimes referred to as field research, hermeneutic, naturalistic inquiry, phenomenological research, symbolic interactionism, descriptive research, interpretive research, and ethnographic studies (Cox & West, 1986; Doehring, 1988; Eastwood, 1988). Qualitative research is non-numerical and involves collection of narrative data about a real life event or situation; in other words, it provides systematic, context-based descriptive data (Plante, Kiernan, & Betts, 1994). Qualitative research is especially well suited to description, hypothesis generation, and theory development (Polit & Hungler, 1991). The primary characteristic of qualitative research is that it is concerned with understanding real-life events or situations. Other characteristics include: (1) it studies a situation or event that can be investigated initially without reference to hypothesis or theory; (2) it allows researcher's subjective point of view into the research; (3) it focuses on a particular setting or situation; (4) its purpose is to clarify the meaning of the event or behavior studied; and (5) it draws on theories or hypotheses as explanations for what is observed (Eastwood, 1988). Qualitative research does not involve quantification of data or statistical analysis and frequently takes the form of a case study (Doehring, 1988; Plante, Kiernan, & Betts, 1994). To clarify qualitative research, characteristics of qualitative and quantitative research are compared in Table 7–2. Cox and West (1986) compared qualitative and quantitative research on the basis of purpose(s), general approach, methodology, and data collection and analysis.

The primary weaknesses of qualitative analysis are related to reliability and validity (Cox & West, 1986). Qualitative analysis lacks objectivity; that is, it is subjective. In research using qualitative analysis, personal biases, viewpoints, and preconceptions about the issues being studied must be searched out and clarified (Eastwood, 1988). Other disadvantages involve difficulties in establishing cause-and-effect relationships; testing research hypotheses; determining opinions, practices and attitudes of a large population; and data analysis. It is extremely time consuming to analyze qualitative, narrative data (Polit & Hungler, 1991).

Qualitative Data Analysis Procedures

Qualitative analysis is challenging because: (1) there are no systematic rules for analyzing and presenting qualitative data, (2) the tremendous amount of work required to organize and analyze narrative data, and (3) reduction of the data for reporting purposes (Polit & Hungler, 1991).

The first step in analyzing qualitative data is organization of the materials. Qualitative data are summarized and organized by

TABLE 7-2. Differences Between Qualitative and Quantitative Research

Characteristic	Qualitative Research	Quantitative Research
Purpose	Understanding	Prediction and control
Reality	Dynamic	Stable
Viewpoint	Insider	Outsider
Values	Value bound	Value free
Focus	Holistic	Particularistic
Orientation	Discovery	Verification
Data	Subjective	Objective
Instrumentation	Human	Nonhuman
Conditions	Naturalistic	Controlled
Results	Valid	Reliable

Source: Adapted from *Understanding and Conducting Qualitative Research* by S. Stainback and W. Stainback, 1988, pp. 8–9. Reston, VA: Council for Exceptional Children.

abstracting the relevant information. After the relevant data are abstracted, several approaches can be used for organizing and summarizing the data such as presenting the data in tabular or narrative form (Silverman, 1993). Analysis of data usually begins with a search for themes or recurring regularities. Sometimes quasi-statistics are used which involve tabulating the frequency with which certain theories or relations occur.

There are specific strategies for analyzing qualitative data: analytic induction, grounded theory, and content analysis. *Analytic induction* involves an interactive approach for analyzing qualitative data by alternating back and forth between tentative explanation for each repetition and gradual refinements and tentative definitions of emerging hypotheses. *Grounded theory* is an approach for analyzing qualitative data through comparison to develop and refine categories. It is more than a method of data analysis because data collection and data analysis occur simultaneously. The purpose of grounded theory is to develop theories and theoretical concepts grounded in real-life observations. A procedure called constant comparison is used to develop and refine theoretically relevant categories (Polit & Hungler, 1991).

Content analysis is a systematic and objective method for quantifying written or verbal data. Data suitable for content analysis include diaries, interviews, journal articles, minutes of meetings, personal reflections, newspaper articles, speeches, audio tapes, and videotapes. There are several units of analysis: themes refer to ideas or concepts, and items refer to the entire message. After the unit of analysis has been selected, a classification system must be developed to permit classification of messages according to content. These coded data can be analyzed statistically or qualitatively (Polit & Hungler, 1991). Aylwin (1988) emphasized the importance of "care in generating the category system so that it arises from the data and not from the researcher's prejudices," and ". . . the use of at least two independent judges to code the data using the category system" (p. 186). Content analysis is systematic because data are methodically included or excluded according to predetermined criteria. It can be used alone or in conjunction with other data collection methods. This technique has the advantages of being expedient and efficient in its use of available materials. It has several disadvantages including the risk of subjectivity and the amount of tedious work involved (Polit & Hungler, 1991). There are a number of publications available about qualitative research: Damico, Maxwell, and Kovarsky (1990), Glaser and Strauss (1967), Kovarsky and Crago (1991), Loflaud and Loflaud (1984), McCall and Simmons (1969), Stainback and Stainback (1988), and Spradley (1979). Several studies of language acquisition have been qualitative and involved diary analyses (Romski, Joyner, & Sevcik, 1987).

A good example of a study implementing qualitative analysis is Schetz and Billingsley (1992). They interviewed 20 school-based speech-language pathologists, asking open-ended questions about administrative support, nonsupport, and solutions for improving support. Responses were summarized on two tables, one listing types of support and the other listing evidence of nonsupport. The lists were arranged according to the frequency each factor was given by the respondents. In discussion of their results, dimensions or categories of support and implications for increasing administrative support for speech-language pathologists were identified.

QUANTITATIVE ANALYSIS: DESCRIPTIVE STATISTICS

Quantitative analysis involves manipulation of numerical data through statistical procedures to describe phenomena or assess the magnitude and reliability of relationships among them (Polit & Hungler, 1991). Graphs and descriptive statistics are used to organize quantitative data. Quantitative and qualitative research are compared in Table 7–2.

Graphs

Several types of graphic displays, including line graphs, bar graphs, pie charts or graphs, and column graphs, can be used to summarize data. Graphs make it easier to inspect and identify trends (Doehring, 1988). To illustrate the possibilities for organizing and summarizing qualitative data, Table 7–3 presents references to representative graphs from articles published in *Asha*.

Descriptive Statistics

Descriptive statistics are used to describe and analyze quantitative data. Raw data that are not organized or analyzed are overwhelming (Polit & Hungler, 1991). It is impossible even to identify general trends until some order or structure is imposed on the data. Consider the 100 numbers presented in Table 7–4. Let us assume that these numbers represent the years of professional experience of 100 speech-language pathologists. Visual inspection of the numbers in this table is not too helpful. The data are too numerous to make much sense of them in this

TABLE 7–3.   References to Representative Graphs Used to Organize and Summarize Qualitative Data in *Asha*

Type of Graph	Volume	Year	Issue	Pages
Histogram or bar graphs	32	1990	(5)	55
	32	1990	(9)	71
	33	1991	(1)	55
	33	1991	(9)	51–53
	35	1993	(1)	64
	35	1993	(4)	42, 47–48
	35	1993	(5)	55
	35	1993	(12)	25
Frequency polygon	32	1990	(5)	55
Smoothed curve polygon	32	1990	(6)	57
Pie chart	35	1993	(6)	59–60

TABLE 7–4. Example of Raw Data Presentation: Years of Experience of 100 Speech-Language Pathologists

27	6	5	10
11	21	15	18
14	14	6	7
10	10	12	13
8	13	7	15
16	9	24	11
12	15	15	10
7	7	13	21
13	12	17	8
9	2	9	14
6	19	14	6
21	11	8	17
11	6	12	11
12	17	16	12
7	12	11	10
5	9	12	22
15	24	15	9
1	4	9	11
4	14	11	10
9	7	12	20
17	12	19	12
10	15	10	13
13	10	13	15
12	13	14	9
20	18	17	16

form. A frequency distribution is one method for organizing and analyzing raw data. Numerical values are ordered from the lowest to the highest with a count of the number of times each value was obtained. The years of experience of the 100 speech-language pathologists are presented as a frequency distribution in Table 7–5. A grouped frequency distribution is shown in Table 7–6. Frequency distributions also can be displayed graphically as a histogram or polygon. A histogram or bar graph is constructed by placing the values on the horizontal axis and then drawing a bar at each value with the height corresponding to the frequency of that value (Bordens & Abbott, 1988; Cox & West, 1986). The frequency polygon uses the same axis as the histogram. It is constructed by placing a dot at the height of each frequency and drawing a straight line to connect the dots. Figures 7–1 through 7–3 show how

TABLE 7–5. Frequency Distribution of Years of Experience of 100 Speech-Language Pathologists

Years of of Experience	Frequency (f)	Percentage (%)
27	1	1
26	0	0
25	0	0
24	2	2
23	0	0
22	1	1
21	3	3
20	2	2
19	3	3
18	2	2
17	5	5
16	3	3
15	7	7
14	6	6
13	8	8
12	12	12
11	8	8
10	10	10
9	8	8
8	3	3
7	6	6
6	5	5
5	2	2
4	2	2
3	0	0
2	1	1
1	0	0
0	0	0
TOTAL	100	100

the same hypothetical data can be presented graphically. Figures 7–1 and 7–2 illustrate the histogram or bar graph and frequency polygon, respectively using the data from Table 7–3. Figure 7–3 illustrates a curve approximating the data in these examples. A set of data can be described relative to the shape of the distribution, central tendency, and variability.

TABLE 7–6. Frequency Distribution of Years of Experience of 100 Speech-Language Pathologists by 5-Year Intervals

Years of Experience	Frequency (f)
25–29	1
20–24	8
15–19	20
10–14	44
5–9	24
0–4	3
TOTAL	100

Distribution

Distribution is the form or shape of numerical values in a sample. A distribution of numerical values can assume an almost endless number of forms or shapes. The most important characteristic of a distribution's shape is its symmetry or modality. A distribution is symmetrical if its two halves are mirror images of one another. These distributions are shown in Figure 7–4. Asymmetrical distributions are usually described as being skewed or non-normal. The peak or high point of the distribution is off-center and one tail is longer than the other. Examples of skewed distributions are illustrated in Figure 7–5. These distributions are usually described relative to the direction of the skew. The distribution is negatively skewed if the longer tail points to the left; that is, most of the values are located at the high end of the frequency distribution. The distribution is positively skewed if the longer tail points toward the right; in other words, a large portion of values are located at the low end. These distributions are said to have ceiling effects and floor effects, respectively. These effects decrease the possibility of demonstrating the effects of independent variables (Doehring, 1988). Skewedness that cannot be identified by visual inspection of a graph may be determined statistically by using the Pearson coefficient of skewness (Bordens & Abbott, 1988).

The *modality of a distribution* is the number of peaks present. A *unimodal distribution* has one peak or high point. A *multimodal distribution* has two or more peaks. The most common type of multimodal distribution is bimodal, a distribution with two peaks or high points. A trimodal distribution has three peaks.

Another descriptive characteristic of distribution is *kurtosis* which describes the flatness or peakedness of the distribution.

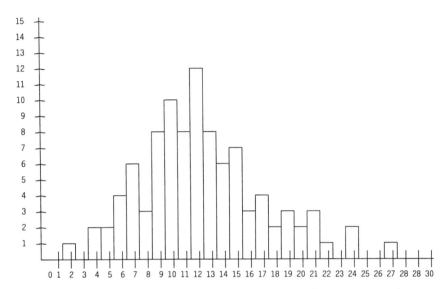

FIGURE 7-1. Histogram Used to Display Years of Experience of 100 Speech-Language Pathologists.

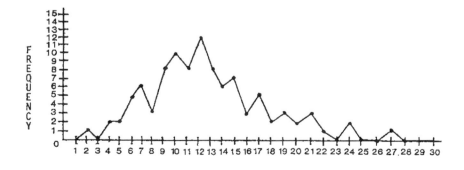

YEARS OF EXPERIENCE

FIGURE 7-2. Frequency Polygon Used to Display Years of Experience of 100 Speech-Language Pathologists.

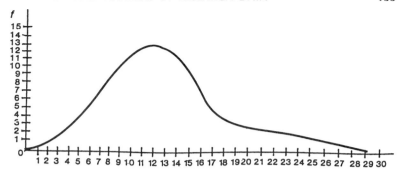

YEARS OF EXPERIENCE

FIGURE 7-3. Smoothed-Curve Used to Display Years of Experience of 100 Speech-language Pathologists.

Flat distributions with long tails are referred to as *platykurtic*; sharply peaked distributions with short tails are referred to as *leptokurtic*. A normal or bell-shaped distribution is symmetrical and unimodal (Cox & West, 1986).

Central Tendency

Measures of central tendency are indexes which represent the average or typical value of a set of numbers. The most commonly used measure of central tendency is the *mean* or simple arithmetic average (Maxfield, Schweitzer, & Gouvier, 1988). It can be computed from measures having interval or ratio properties (Silverman, 1993). The mean is usually the preferred measure of central tendency because it is the easiest to compute and is useful in further statistical analysis (Polit & Hungler, 1991; Silverman, 1993). It is obtained by adding all values and dividing by the number of values used to obtain the total.

The *median* is the midpoint of a set of values, that is, the halfway value. It can be computed from measures having interval, ordinal, or ratio properties (Silverman, 1993). The median is the most appropriate measure of central tendency for skewed, asymmetric data (Isaac & Michael, 1987; Maxfield et al., 1988). The *mode*, or most frequently occurring value in a distribution, is not used very often because data usually do not have a single, clearly defined mode. It is appropriate for measures having interval, nominal, ordinal, or ratio properties (Silverman, 1993). The mode is used as a quick estimate of central

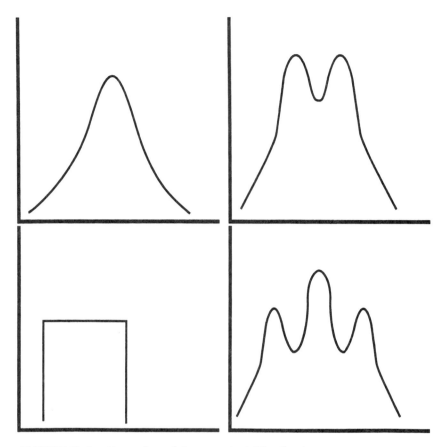

FIGURE 7–4.   Examples of Symmetrical Distributions.

value and to identify the most typical case (Isaac & Michael, 1987). Silverman (1993) considers the mode as a less stable and reliable measure of central tendency than the mean or median.

Variability

Variability is the spread or dispersion of the data. Measures of variability are the standard deviation (SD), the range, and the semi-interquartile range (Q). The most commonly used measure of variability is the standard deviation. The *standard deviation* is a variability measure of the degree to which each value deviates from the mean. This measure of the degree of variability in a set of scores is relatively easy to

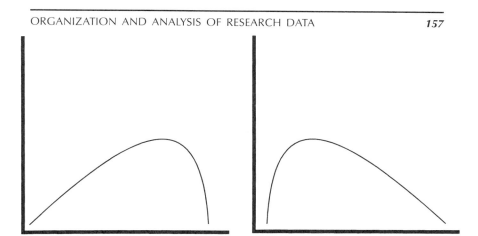

Negative Skew   Positive Skew

FIGURE 7–5.   Examples of Skewed Distributions

compute and is obtained by first calculating deviation scores, which represent the degree to which each value deviates from the mean. It is an appropriate index of variability for measures having interval or ratio properties (Silverman, 1993). The SD is relatively easy to interpret and is useful in further statistical analysis. Its value is less likely to be distorted by a few extreme measures although it can be misleading for skewed data (Maxfield et al., 1988).

In a normal or bell-shaped distribution that is symmetric and unimodal, the standard deviation is a useful characteristic in considering some inferential statistical techniques (Cox & West, 1986). Three standard deviations below and above the mean include practically all values (99%) in a normal distribution (see Figure 7–6). The area between the mean and either -1 or +1 standard deviation is equal to 34.1% of the total area. Thus, about 68% of all values fall within ±1 standard deviation of the mean. The area between the mean and either +2 or –2 standard deviations is equal to 47.7% of the total area. Therefore, approximately 95% fall within ± 2 standard deviations of the mean. In a normal distribution, the mean, median, and mode are the same.

The *range* is the distance between the lowest and highest values in the distribution. The larger the range the more variability there is in a distribution; conversely, the smaller the range, the less variability there is in a distribution (Ventry & Schiavetti, 1986). It is an appropriate index of variability for measures having interval, ordinal, or ratio properties (Silverman, 1993). The range is relatively easy to compute and interpret, and is useful if information about extreme scores is wanted (Isaac & Michael, 1987).

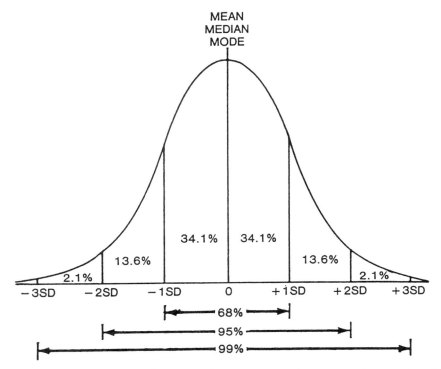

FIGURE 7-6. Normal Curve Characteristics. (From *Fundamentals of Research for Health Professionals* by R. C. Cox and W. L. West, 1986, p. 78. Rockville, MD: American Occupational Therapy Foundation, Inc., with permission. Copyright 1986 American Occupational Therapy Foundation, Inc.)

The *semi-interquartile range* (Q) indicates half of the range of values within which the middle 50% of the values lie. In other words, it is the interval between the first and third quartiles. It is an appropriate index of variability for measures having interval, ordinal, or ratio properties (Silverman, 1993). The semi-interquartile range is appropriate for measuring variability when there is extreme skewing. It is, however, not as easy to interpret as the range (Silverman, 1993).

Relationships Among Variables

Correlation coefficients are statistics that summarize the strength and direction of the relationship between two variables (Bordens & Abbott, 1988; Polit & Hungler, 1991; Silverman, 1993). The most common measure of correlation is the Pearson product-moment correlation co-efficient which is sometimes referred to as Pearson's r. The values of the correlation coefficient range from -1.00 for a perfect negative correlation, through 0.0 for no relationship, to $+1.00$ for a perfect positive correlation. The larger the correlation coefficient plus or minus 1, the stronger the relationship. A *negative correlation* is an inverse relationship in which a high value of one variable is associated with low values of the other variable. A *positive correlation* is a direct relationship in which two measures increase or decrease together. The Pearson r is appropriate for measures having interval or ratio properties (Bordens & Abbott, 1988).

In a study comparing metaphoric comprehension in normal, traumatic brain injured (TBI), and language learning disabled (LLD) adolescents, Towne and Entwisle (1993) did Pearson r correlations to compare the age of the subjects in each group and their performances on the metaphoric subtest. Correlation coefficients were not statistically significant at a confidence level of $p < .05$ when comparing age and test performance in any of the groups. Thus, it was concluded that the difference in performance among the groups was not related to age.

Correlation data can be plotted on a two-dimensional graph called a scatter plot, scatter diagram, or scattergram to graphically display the relationship between two variables. To construct a scatter plot, a scale for two variables is constructed at right angles, making a rectangle-coordinate graph (Polit & Hungler, 1991). The range of values for the variable (X) is scaled off along the horizontal axis, and the same is done for the second variable (Y) along the vertical axis. Each pair of scores is represented as a point on the graph. The direction of the slope indicates the direction of the correlation. If the slope of points begins at the lower left corner and extends to the upper right corner, the relationship is positive. The relationship is negative if the slope of points begins at the lower right corner and extends to the upper left corner. Scattergrams of correlations of different strengths are shown in Figure 7–7. Other less frequently used measures of correlation are the point biserial correlation, Spearman's rho, and the phi coefficient (Bordens & Abbott, 1988).

INTEGRATION OF QUALITATIVE AND QUANTITATIVE ANALYSIS

Research could be enhanced by collection and integration of both qualitative and quantitative data. Plante, Kiernan, and Betts (1994) state that "qualitative and quantitative methods are both capable of providing

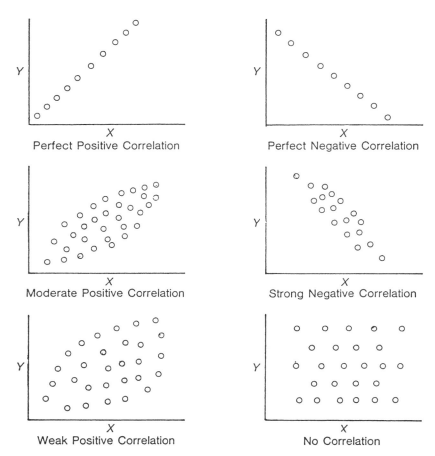

FIGURE 7-7. Scattergrams of Correlations of Different Strengths. (From *Fundamentals of Research for Health Professionals* by R. C. Cox and W. L. West, 1986, p. 74. Rockville, MD: American Occupational Therapy Foundation, Inc., with permission. Copyright 1986 American Occupational Therapy Foundation, Inc.)

scientifically important and clinically relevant information" (p. 52). Stainback and Stainback (1988) suggest that combining qualitative and quantitative research is advantageous. Cox and West (1986) believe that the two approaches "compliment each other quite well" (p. 50).

The integration of both types of data has several advantages including complementary strengths and weaknesses, enhanced theoretical insights, multiple feedback loops which add to the incremental gains in knowledge, enhanced validity, and further study when there are inconsistent findings (Polit & Hungler, 1991). There are also disadvantages such as epistemological biases; high costs; inadequate training of researchers, because most graduate level training stresses either qualitative or quantitative research; and publication bias. Some journals prefer qualitative studies, while others prefer studies that are quantitative (Polit & Hungler, 1991).

Qualitative and quantitative research can be integrated in several ways (Polit & Hungler, 1991). One strategy is to collect both qualitative and quantitative data within the context of an experimental or quasi-experimental study. A second strategy is to combine structured data collection with fieldwork. A third strategy is to include qualitative methods within a survey. Figure 7–8 illustrates strategies for integrating qualitative and quantitative methods. Note that the third strategy is the reverse of the second strategy in that quantitative findings are used to help explain qualitative results (Steckler et al., 1992).

INFERENTIAL STATISTICS

Inferential statistics provide a way to make inferences about a population based on data obtained in a sample (Polit & Hungler, 1991). These statistics test hypotheses by drawing inferences or generalizations from small groups to larger groups. The variability of scores within each group (the within-group variance) is compared with the variability of measures between groups or the between-group variance (Bordens & Abbott, 1988). According to Silverman (1993), inferential statistics can provide answers to several kinds of questions about a set of data: (1) reliability of differences or relationships observed in a set of data; (2) generality of differences and relationships observed in a set of data; (3) population values, or magnitudes, of descriptive statistics and of differences between descriptive statistics; and (4) inferences about factors that influence a particular judgment or performance on a particular task or more reliably distinguish between groups.

Sample statistics contain a certain degree of error as estimates of population parameters. Inferential statistics provide a means for deciding whether the sampling error is too high to provide reliable population estimates (Polit & Hungler, 1991). The sampling distribution of the mean is the distribution of the means of many different samples drawn from the same population. The sampling distribution of the mean follows a normal distribution or curve, and is the same as the mean of the population from which the samples were drawn (Bordens & Abbott, 1988). The standard error of the measurement (SEM) is used to estimate the standard deviation of the sampling distribution of the mean

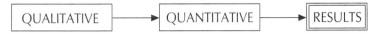

1. Qualitative methods are used to help develop quantitative measures.

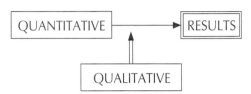

2. Qualitative methods are used to help explain quantitative findings.

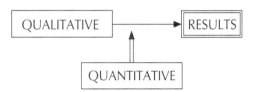

3. Quantitative methods are used to help explain qualitative findings.

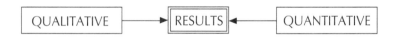

4. Qualitative and quantitative methods are used equally.

FIGURE 7–8. Strategies for Integrating Qualitative and Quantitative Methods. (From "Toward Integrating Qualitative and Quantitative Methods: An Introduction" by A. Steckler, K. R. McLeroy, R. M. Goodman, S. T. Bird, and L. McCormick, 1992. *Health Education Quarterly, 19*(1), 108, with permission. Copyright 1992 John Wiley & Sons.)

of the population from which the sample was drawn. The smaller the standard error of the measurement, the more accurate are the estimates of the population value.

Statistical inference consists of two approaches: (1) estimating parameters and (2) testing hypotheses. The value of an unknown population characteristic can be estimated by means of point or interval estimation. Point estimation provides a single numerical value. Interval estimation, which is sometimes referred to as confidence intervals, provides the upper and lower limits of a range of values between which the population value is expected to fall at some specified probability level.

Inferential statistics make it possible to make a decision about the validity of the null hypothesis while controlling the probability of incorrectly rejecting the null hypothesis. This is a *Type I, or alpha, error* (Bordens & Abbott, 1988). A Type I error can occur for several reasons: (1) on the basis of random fluctuation there is a large enough difference or relationship for a null hypothesis to be rejected, and (2) biased measures related to preconceived expectations about the results of the research (Silverman, 1993). The *null hypothesis* is a statement that there is no relationship between the variables and that any observed relationships result from chance or sampling fluctuations (Polit & Hungler, 1991; Silverman, 1993). Failure to reject the null hypothesis means that any observed differences are attributable to chance fluctuation. If a null hypothesis is not rejected when it should be, a *Type II, or beta, error* occurs.

Type I errors can be minimized by establishing levels of significance. A *level of significance* or alpha level represents the probability of making a Type I error. Type I errors are less likely if the level of significance or alpha is smaller. The two most frequently used levels of significance are .01 and .05 which means there is a 1 % and 5 % probability of a null hypothesis being true.

Ottenbacher and Barrett (1990) reviewed 100 data-based rehabilitation studies and reported "the possibility of a high rate of Type II errors which represent a false-negative conclusion" (p. 102). In other words, a null hypothesis that was false was accepted when it should have been rejected. The Bonferroni method is a procedure for reducing Type I errors, but it can be overly conservative and result in a loss of statistical power when a small number of comparisons are evaluated. Ottenbacher (1991) suggests a modification of the Bonferroni which allows the control of Type I errors but maintains statistical power.

For example, Cole, Mills, and Kelley (1994) administered tests of cognitive skills and language skills to young children in an effort to determine the level of agreement among the tests used to identify delays in language and cognitive skills. The level of agreement among the three cognitive measures using a repeated measures analysis of variance revealed significant ($p < .05$) differences among the test scores. To examine the differences among the test scores, t-tests were done using the Bonferroni adjustment for Type I error. Significant differences in all three possible pairs of cognitive test scores were found.

The same analysis was done to study the relationship among the four language measures. Repeated measures analysis of variance determined a significant difference among all measures ($p < .05$). However, t-tests to compare the six possible combinations of the four tests using the Bonferroni adjustment revealed only two significant differences ($p < .05$). Thus, four of the pairs were not significantly different, as would have been concluded by looking only at the repeated measures analysis of variance.

Muma (1993) reviewed studies published in the *Journal of Speech and Hearing Disorders* and *Journal of Speech and Hearing Research.* Ten issues from 1979 to 1989 from each journal were randomly sampled. Based on the probabilities of Type I and Type II errors, there are likely to be about 50 to 250 false findings. Replication provides verification and disconfirmation; however, there were only 12 replications in the studies Muma reviewed. More recently, Silverman and Marik (1993) and Ingham, Cordes, and Finn (1993) replicated earlier studies. There is an obvious need for more replication of studies.

Type IV errors are a variation of Type I errors. Type IV errors result from incorrect interpretation of a correctly rejected hypothesis. These errors usually result from misinterpretation of the data rather than from incorrect application of a statistical test (Ottenbacher, 1992).

Statistical significance indicates that the results obtained are probably not caused by chance. Two features contribute to statistical significance: (1) the size of the difference between means and (2) the variability among values. In most hypothesis testing, *two-tailed tests* are used in which both ends or tails of the sampling distribution are used to determine the range of improbable values. One-tailed tests are controversial and used infrequently. A one-tailed test may be used if there is a strong logical or theoretical reason for a directional hypothesis and for assuming that findings opposite to the direction hypothesized are virtually impossible (Polit & Hungler, 1991). According to Silverman (1993) "it is advantageous to use a one-tailed test if it is appropriate to do so because the probability of committing a Type II error is less than for a two-tailed test" (p. 211).

The two types of inferential statistics are nonparametric and parametric. *Nonparametric statistics* are inferential statistics that do not involve vigorous assumptions about the population from which the sample was drawn. They are sometimes referred to as distribution-free statistics because assumptions about the distribution of the critical variables are less restrictive. Nonparametric statistics have the advantages of speed and ease of computations, and appropriateness for studies that yield outcomes that are difficult to quantify. Disadvantages include

reduced efficiency, less specific hypothesis testing, and failure to utilize all of the special characteristics of a distribution (Kuzma, 1984).
This type of statistic is appropriate for nominal and ordinal scales (Polit
& Hungler, 1991). Nonparametric tests include the chi square test (X^2),
the Mann-Whitney U test, the median test, the sign test, the Wilcoxin
signed rank test, and the Kruskal-Wallis and Friedman tests. Description of these and other statistical methods are presented in Table 7–7.
There are also several other nonparametric tests (Bordens & Abbott,
1988). The most frequently used nonparametric test is the chi square
X^2 which is designed for frequency data in which the relationship or
contingency between two variables is to be determined.

In a study of the ability of teachers to accurately identify disordered voices, Davis and Harris (1992) used nonparametric statistical
tests because the data were collected in categories. Trained teachers'
judgments and untrained student education majors' judgments in identifying normal and abnormal voices and designating whether referral
was appropriate were designated to four categories for each group. Chi
square was used to compare the teacher and student data categories.
Results indicated the teachers and students categorized normal and
abnormal voices correctly more than chance would allow. However,
teachers more frequently appropriately judged that referral was appropriate than did the students.

Parametric statistics are inferential statistics that involve making
assumptions about the parametrics of the population from which the
research sample was drawn. Parametric statistics involve: (1) assumptions about the distribution of variables and (2) the estimation of at least
one parameter. They are appropriate statistics for interval and ordinal
scales. Parametric statistics are usually preferred because they are more
powerful and are more likely to reject a null hypothesis that is not true.
The most common parametric statistics are the *t*-test and analysis of
variance (ANOVA) (see Table 7–7). The *t*-test, sometimes referred to as
student's *t*, can handle only two group situations. There are several special versions of the *t*-test for between-subjects and within-subjects designs
(Bordens & Abbott, 1988). ANOVA can be applied to three or more
groups, as well as to more than one independent variable. The statistic
used in ANOVA to determine statistical significance is the F-ratio which
is the ratio of between-groups variability to within-group variability.

Statistical or bivariate tests used to analyze the significance of the
relationship between two variables simultaneously include Pearson's *r*
for interval measures, Spearman's rho and Kendall's tau for ordinal
measures, and the phi coefficient and Cramer's V for nominal measures
(Polit & Hungler, 1991).

TABLE 7-7. Description of Statistical Methods

Method	Description
Nonparametric	
Chi-square	Used to assess whether a relationship exists between two nominal level variables.
Cramer's V	Index which describes the magnitude of relationship between nominal level data.
Fisher's exact test	Used to test the significance of the differences in properties.
Friedman test	Used with paired groups on a repeated measures situation to test for analysis of variance by ranks.
Kendall's tau	Correlation coefficient used to indicate the magnitude of a relationship between ordinal level data.
Kruskal-Wallis test	Used to test the difference between three or more independent groups based on ranked scores.
Mann-Whitney U test	Used to test the difference between two independent groups, based on ranked scores.
McNeman test	Compares differences in proportions, when values are derived from paired, nonindependent groups.
Median test	Compares median values of two independent groups to determine if groups derive from populations with different medians.
Phi coefficient	Index that describes the magnitude of relationship between two dichotomous variables.
Spearman's rho	Correlation coefficient that indicates magnitude of relationship between variables measured on ordinal scale.

TABLE 7–7. *(continued)*

Method	Description
Wilcoxin signed rank test	Compares two paired groups, based on relative ranking of values between pairs.
Parametric	
ANOVA	Tests effect of one or more treatments on different groups by comparing variability between groups to variability within groups.
Pearson *r*	Designates magnitude of relationship between two variables measured on interval or ordinal scales.
t test	Used for analyzing the difference between two means.

Source: Adapted from *Nursing Research: Principles and Methods* by D. F. Polit and B. P. Hungler, 1991. Philadelphia: J. B. Lippincott.

ADVANCED STATISTICAL PROCEDURES

Multivariate tests are used to study the relationship among three or more variables. Currently, these techniques are being used more often than the traditional approach to data analysis and research design consisting of studying the effect of a single independent variable or a single dependent variable. Multivariate techniques are designed to analyze the relationship among three or more variables (Buchner & Findley, 1990). Multivariate techniques have been widely used in recent years because of the increased computing capabilities of computers (Isaac & Michael, 1987). Polit and Hungler (1991) believe that both consumers and producers of research are at a strong disadvantage if they are not familiar with multivariate procedures. Multivariate procedures include analysis of covariance, discriminate analysis, factor analysis, multiple regression, path analysis, and power analysis. Table 7–8 provides a brief description of these procedures.

For example, Saniga and Carlin (1993) studied responses of parents of children in kindergarten through second grade to the Voice Conservation Index (a questionnaire about vocal habits). Multivariate analysis of variance (MANOVA) was used to examine the effect of age

TABLE 7-8. Description of Multivariate Statistical Methods

Method	Description
Analysis of covariance	Tests effect of one or more treatments on different groups while controlling for one or more extraneous variables (covariates).
Discriminate analysis	Used to predict group membership or status on a categorial (nominal level) variable on the basis of two or more independent variables.
Factor analysis	Reduces a large set of variables into a smaller set of variables with common characteristics or underlying dimensions.
Multiple regression	Procedure for understanding the simultaneous effects of two or more independent (or extraneous) variables on a dependent variable; the dependent variable must be measured on an interval or ratio scale.
Path analysis	Regression-based procedure for testing causal methods, usually involves nonexperimental data.
Power analysis	Procedure for estimating the likelihood of committing a Type II error or sample size requirements.

Source: Adapted from *Nursing Research: Principles and Methods* by D. F. Polit and B. P. Hungler, 1991, Philadelphia: J. B. Lippincott.

of the children on the parents' perception of 16 vocal behaviors. It was determined that the parents of younger children perceived vocal behaviors differently than parents of older children.

SUMMARY

This chapter concentrated on the organization and analysis of research data in speech-language pathology and audiology research. Stages of data management include methods for (1) data entry, (2) preliminary data analysis, (3) primary data analysis, and (4) secondary data analysis.

Data may be examined using the following: qualitative analysis, quantitative analysis, and integration of qualitative and quantitative analysis. Several types of graphic displays which make it easier to identify trends from the data were discussed and illustrated.

Descriptive statistics include measures of central tendency (mean, median, and mode) and variability (standard deviation, range of values in total or in quartiles). Procedures for preventing a Type I Error (incorrectly rejecting a null hypothesis) or a Type II Error (accepting a null hypothesis that is false) were discussed. Statistical procedures between two variables and advanced multivariate statistical procedures for determining the relationship among three or more variables were discussed and/or presented in tables.

STUDY EXERCISES

1. Give an example of the clinical use of qualitative and of quantitative data.

2. What are the basic principles that apply to all stages of data management?

3. What are the stages of data management?

4. Differentiate between qualitative and quantitative analysis.

5. How do analysis techniques for qualitative (categorical) data compare with those for quantitative data?

6. What is the difference between descriptive and inferential statistics?

7. What are the divisions of inferential statistics?

8. Review the articles you and your team have already reviewed for other exercises. Have any of the authors implemented the use of graphic display of data? If so, what type(s)? Did the graphs clearly convey information about the data?

9. What do the mean, median, and mode have in common? How do they differ?

10. What is variability? Name and explain the measures of variability.

11. How are relationships between two variables graphically displayed? What statistical tests may be used to determine significance of relationship between two variables?

12. In what three ways might a researcher integrate qualitative and quantitative research?

13. Explain the purpose of and procedure (point estimation and confidence interval estimation) for estimating parameters.

14. Explain hypothesis testing. What types of errors might be made when testing hypotheses? How might these errors be avoided?

15. Explain how establishing a level of significance, or alpha level, affects hypothesis testing.

16. What is the difference between parametric and nonparametric statistics?

17. It is important to remember that statistical techniques do not think for you. Give an example in which you believe the statistical techniques would indicate a difference between two groups that you would not consider to be important or meaningful.

18. You developed a research question, a procedure for sampling a population, and developed a data collection form for Exercises 5, 6, 8, and 10 in Chapter 6. Answer the following questions as a continuation of that project.

a. How will data be categorized?

b. How will reliability and validity be established?

c. What statistical measure(s) would be appropriate?

d. How will the data be displayed?

19. What should a researcher know about a statistical method before using it?

20. Why is a statistician an important member of a research team?

21. Use the checklist (Table 7–1) to assess statistical aspects of the findings of three papers published in the *Journal of Speech and Hearing Research*. You may have already reviewed at least some papers from this journal in Exercise 8.

SUGGESTED READINGS

Bordens, K. S., & Abbott, B. B. (1988). *Research designs and methods.* Mountain View, CA: Mayfield. Chapter 11, Describing data, pp. 293–326. Chapter 12, Using inferential statistics, pp. 327–361. Chapter 13, Using the computer to analyze data, pp. 362–393.

Buchner, D. M., & Findley, T. W. (1990). Research in physical medicine and rehabilitation VIII: Preliminary data analysis. *American Journal of Physical Medicine and Rehabilitation, 69*(3), 154–168.

Denson, T. (1986). Organization and analysis of data. In I. M. Ventry & N. Schiavetti: (Eds.), *Evaluation research in speech pathology and audiology* (pp. 143–188). New York: MacMillan.

Feigal, D., Black, D., Hearst, N., Grady, D., Fox, C., Newman, T. B., & Hulley, S. B. (1988). Planning for data management and analysis. In S. B. Hulley & S. R. Cummings (Eds.), *Designing clinical research* (pp. 159–171). Baltimore, MD: Williams & Wilkins.

Findley, T. W. (1990). Research in physical medicine and rehabilitation IX: Primary data analysis. *American Journal of Physical Medicine and Rehabilitation, 69*(4), 208–218.

Findley, T. W., & Stineman, M. G. (1989). Research in physical medicine and rehabilitation V: Data entry and early exploratory data analysis. *American Journal of Physical Medicine and Rehabilitation, 68*(5), 240–251.

Huck, S. W., Cormier, W. H., & Bounds, W. G. (1974). *Reading statistics and research.* New York: HarperCollins. Chapter 3, Introduction to inferential statistics, pp. 38–48. Chapter 4, t tests, one-way analysis of variance and multiple comparison procedures, pp. 49–73. Chapter 5, Factorial analyses of variates. pp. 74–102. Chapter 6, Analysis of variance with repeated measures, pp. 103–131. Chapter 7, The analysis of covariance, pp. 132–147. Chapter 8, Multiple correlation and discriminate function analysis, pp. 148–176. Chapter 9, Multivariate analogs to the t test, the analysis of variance, and the analysis of covariance, pp. 177–195. Chapter 10, Nonparametric statistical tests, pp. 196–221.

Isaac, S., & Michael, W. B. (1987). *Handbook in research and evaluation,* San Diego, CA: Edits Publishers, Chapter 5, Statistical techniques and the analysis of data, pp. 157–206.

Kuzma, J. W. (1984). *Basic statistics for the health sciences.* Mountain View, CA: Mayfield.

McAleer, S. (1990). Twelve tips for using statistics. *Medical Teacher, 12*(2), 127–130.

Polit, D. F., & Hungler, B. P. (1991). *Nursing research: Principles and methods.* Philadelphia: J. B. Lippincott. Part V: The analysis of research data, pp. 403–562.

Silverman, F. H. (1993). *Research design and evaluation in speech-language pathology and audiology.* Englewood Cliffs, NJ: Prentice-Hall. Chapter 9, Organizing data for answering questions: Description techniques, pp. 165–198. Chapter 10, Organizing data for answering questions: Inferential techniques, pp. 199–226.

CHAPTER 8

UTILIZATION OF COMMUNICATION DISORDERS RESEARCH

GRACE F. MIDDLETON

- Research Utilization in Communication Disorders
- Barriers to Utilizing Research in Communication Disorders
- Responsibility for Research Utilization
- Summary
- Study Exercises
- Suggested Readings

Research in communication disorders appears in professional journals; is presented at workshops, seminars, and conventions; and is summarized and taught in university courses in speech-language pathology and audiology. Also, small clusters of individuals may share findings as they research topics of special interest. Thus, research in communication disorders is readily available to speech-language pathologists and audiologists. It is the responsibility of every practicing professional to remain updated in order to comply with the ASHA Code of Ethics which provides that the welfare of those served must be held paramount.

RESEARCH UTILIZATION IN
COMMUNICATION DISORDERS

Research is generally utilized by individuals (1) seeking to improve their clinical skills and management techniques; (2) interested in doing research and aspiring to improve their research skills; and (3) using the research to reference information taught to students (Findley, 1989). A fringe benefit of studying the research for any of these purposes is that readers become more informed consumers of research and may become more confident as potential researchers. Fortunately, the current trend is to consider the reader or consumer of research and to present studies in formats that will be easily understood by the targeted readership (Findley, 1989).

Research in communication disorders may be utilized to improve the quality of clinical management. For example, application of research methodology may contribute to the improvement of clinically used scales such as the *Patient Evaluation and Conference System* (PECS) scales used in rehabilitation programs for determining patient progress. Silverstein and associates (1992) analyzed 5500 PECS assessments to identify areas where the scales could be improved, particularly in the sequencing of skills on a continuum according to difficulty. Similar studies may facilitate the improvement of numerous such scales (e.g., coma scales, global measures, disability measures, measures of cognitive ability, and measures of communication function) used for diagnosis and treatment planning by various disciplines including speech-language pathology (Johnston, Findley, DeLuca, & Katz, 1991).

A major consideration in selecting a quality graduate program in communication disorders is the research component provided by the program. The expectation that students who graduate with the master's degree in communication disorders will be ready to do research independently may be unrealistic. However, graduates of a quality master's program should be intelligent consumers of research. They should be able to (1) read and understand the research published in professional journals; (2) apply the information to clinical practice; and (3) appreciate the fact that the origin of the scales, tests, and clinical management programs used daily in clinical practice originated as research projects (Siegel, 1991–1992). Regardless of their exposure to energetic lectures in graduate classes about the importance of being a consumer of research, practicing clinicians seem eventually to "join the chorus of complaints that the journals are not really relevant to their needs, that the articles are too esoteric and technical to be understood, and that they are too dull to be endured" (Siegel, 1991–1992, p. 87).

Of course, as Siegel further points out, much of the published research may not be relevant to daily clinical activity. However, it is the seasoned, knowledgeable clinician who is best suited for the task of gleaning useful clinical knowledge from the available research. Those who are astute consumers of research are able to apply research findings to clinical practice, thus making the most recent discoveries available to clients receiving clinical services.

To become knowledgeable consumers of research, students need hands-on practice doing research. Graduate students need to undertake small, narrowly defined research projects and complete them. The projects should follow simple research designs and should be completed despite errors that occur in the experiment. These should be considered learning experiences, not obstacles to the completion of the study. After all, clinical research is difficult to design, control, and interpret even for the most seasoned researcher(s) (Siegel, 1991–1992).

For those who are interested in doing research and improving their skills, becoming an astute consumer of research is the first step. Finding a published mentor or an experienced research team to collaborate with is an efficient way to begin a lifetime involvement in doing research.

BARRIERS TO UTILIZING RESEARCH IN COMMUNICATION DISORDERS

As enrollments increase in graduate programs in communication disorders, time pressures and budgetary constraints may limit the opportunity for master's level graduate students to conduct independent research. As Siegel (1991–1992, p. 87) pointed out, "the thesis is fast becoming an endangered form." This is unfortunate because the thesis offers the best opportunity for students to practice and develop skills for consuming and conducting research. Furthermore, graduate faculty may tend to discourage students from doing theses because they divert faculty energies away from their own research projects (Siegel, 1991–1992). A research setting with available subjects and cooperative staff is also needed for students to conduct graduate research (Lieske, 1986). Such settings must be identified and the projects coordinated by faculty members who are informed about the requirements and procedures for conducting research by the facility.

Graduate students in some communication disorders programs do not receive adequate instruction in research methods because of the lack of available faculty who are experienced and actively conducting research (Boice & Jones, 1984). Faculty are expected to serve on numerous university, college, and departmental committees, and many are heavily involved in administrative activities in addition to teaching. Furthermore, some are attracted by the immediate rewards of contracting their services. Thus, time constraints and limited interest in the tedium of conducting research may contribute to a decrease in the number of faculty actively involved in research.

To become effective consumers of research, students need a broad knowledge base including (1) knowledge of the subject matter including the technical vocabulary and theoretical concepts, (2) knowledge of research methods including the technical aspects that may not be explained in journal articles, (3) experience reading articles, and (4) practice in evaluating research reports (Hegde, 1994). Hegde (1994) provides an outline to guide the student conducting an evaluation of a research report (see Table 8–1). However, he cautions the reader about the importance of being a critical, not cynical, reviewer while maintaining enthusiasm for research.

For those who are experienced consumers of research and who have had opportunities to conduct research while in graduate training, time constraints may still impede the service provider in utilizing available research. Furthermore, mentors who are actively involved in research may not be readily available to those engaged in clinical practice. Some rehabilitation hospitals interested in clinical management efficacy research may be willing to negotiate a specified number of hours each week for staff to engage in research projects. Some may even be willing to hire a consultant to help the staff set up research projects. Regardless, individuals should be willing to designate part of their discretionary time to do research.

Clinical efficacy research provides the opportunity to develop an on-site research team (Findley & DeLisa, 1990). Such a team effort may break down some of the barriers to doing research in the clinical setting by distributing the work among several individuals and utilizing the research expertise of all members. Furthermore, active involvement

TABLE 8-1. Checklist for Evaluating a Research Report

	Adequate	Inadequate
Significance of the problem investigated	☐	☐
Introduction and literature review		
Clear and complete	☐	☐
Objective, impartial, appropriately critical	☐	☐
Provided purpose for the present study	☐	☐
Statement of the problem		
Clear, replicable	☐	☐
Clear hypotheses or research questions	☐	☐
Methods		
Clear, adequate, replicable	☐	☐
Subject selection, treatment clear and appropriate	☐	☐
Research design readily understood	☐	☐
Research design appropriate and correctly implemented	☐	☐
Results		
Stated unambiguously, objectively	☐	☐
Appropriate method of data analysis	☐	☐
Appropriate use of statistical procedures	☐	☐
Figures and tables used effectively	☐	☐
Data presentation orderly/logical	☐	☐
Discussion		
Results discussed adequately	☐	☐
Hypotheses rejected appropriately or research questions answered	☐	☐
Findings related to previous studies	☐	☐
Implications of the study included	☐	☐

(continued)

TABLE 8–1. *(continued)*

	Adequate	Inadequate
Discussion *(continued)*		
Suggestions included for additional research	☐	☐
Limitations of study discussed	☐	☐
References		
Included only works cited in text	☐	☐
Accurate and in correct format	☐	☐
Appendix		
Necessary to understanding of report	☐	☐
Appropriate or sufficient in length	☐	☐

Source: Adapted from *Clinical Research in Communicative Disorders: Principles and Strategies* by M. N. Hegde, 1994. Austin, TX: Pro-Ed.

in such projects may increase self-confidence of the team members, improve staff morale, and most importantly, improve clinical services.

In addition to limited knowledge and time constraints, an additional barrier to utilizing research exists in the research itself. Replication of studies in an effort to apply the findings to varied populations may occur only over a long period of time. Also, flaws often are readily identified in individual studies. Therefore, the implementation of procedures suggested by research may take years due to the reluctance to change procedures until the research provides indisputable evidence to support the change (Polit & Hungler, 1991). A vicious cycle ensues. On the one hand, busy practitioners await adequate evidence to support change in clinical procedures. On the other hand, there are not enough clinical researchers to replicate needed studies. It is evident that increased numbers of practicing clinicians need to provide the data to substantiate the effectiveness of clinical management programming already in use and to determine the changes needed in clinical management programming that has not proven effective.

RESPONSIBILITY FOR RESEARCH UTILIZATION

Researchers have the responsibility of doing projects that can more readily be utilized. This can be done by doing quality research, planning replications of studies to confirm results, collaborating with clinicians to determine their needs, and reporting the results expeditiously and to large numbers of clinicians even if it means rewriting and resubmitting manuscripts until they are accepted. Furthermore, researchers have a responsibility to present findings at conventions, seminars, and workshops. Research articles should be written clearly and the data presented in a readily understandable format so that consumers will find them more user friendly. Furthermore, the discussion of research findings should include clinical implications of the findings (Polit & Hungler, 1991).

Scholars and educators also have a responsibility to use research. They must incorporate research findings into the curriculum. Students should not just be taught facts and procedures. They need to understand the research on which those facts and procedures are based. Educators also need to be strong role models for students by sharing the findings of their own research and by conveying positive attitudes toward the importance of research to the profession. Students must be taught how to evaluate, summarize, and compare available research on a specific topic. Planning a research project is also excellent experience for students (Polit & Hungler, 1991).

Practicing clinicians have the responsibility of reading widely and critically on topics relevant to their clinical practice. Attendance at professional conferences provides clinicians with the opportunity to learn about research findings that may not be available in print due to the lag time involved in reviewing, rewriting, resubmitting and publishing an article. Clinicians should not accept practices as effective just because they have been used for a long time. Quality clinical practice includes the collection of continued evidence to support the effectiveness of preferred and employed methods. When seeking employment, speech-language pathologists and audiologists who wish to fully utilize research findings in clinical practice and/or to do research, might consider the flexibility the facility seems willing to grant in support of such endeavors (Polit & Hungler, 1991).

Clinicians also may become involved in journal groups that meet regularly to critically review and discuss clinical applications of research articles targeted by the group. In addition, clinicians need to be willing to assist in the collection of data for a project already under way. Participation in such institutional projects is an excellent way to develop improved skills as a researcher and as a consumer of research (Polit & Hungler, 1991).

The facility administrator(s), supervisors, and department chairs also have a responsibility for the utilization of research. An administration that is resistant to change does not provide a climate that encourages intellectual curiosity, critical thinking, and open communication.

Certainly if the administration of a facility is not supportive, the time, continuing education, and financial and resource support needed to conduct projects will not be available. Involvement of administrators in projects and rewarded efforts for doing research or making innovative changes in procedure based on current findings often lead to increased display of administrative support for utilizing and conducting research (Polit & Hungler, 1991).

When the clinical environment is conducive to innovation and study, clinical questions may be raised and researched using a literature review (Lieske,1986). If answers are not evident from the available research, an original study may be undertaken to create a knowledge base on the topic. Most such studies are undertaken if they appear to have clinical relevance, scientific merit, and potential for implementation given the available number of subjects and the feasibility of the study based on available resources (Polit & Hungler, 1991).

It is the responsibility of university faculty and practicing clinicians to pursue adequate funding for research projects and to develop "mentorships" for beginning researchers (Lieske, 1986). In so doing, larger databases and multiple data collection studies can be undertaken, thus increasing the stature of communication disorders in the scientific community.

SUMMARY

Research in communication disorders is readily available to speech-language pathologists and audiologists. It is generally utilized by clinicians to improve the quality of clinical management and by faculty to reference information taught to students. Barriers to utilizing research include limited experience doing research in graduate school, a scarcity of mentors and research teams with whom to collaborate on projects, and limited time and resources for research activities in clinical settings. The responsibility for research utilization lies with the researchers already conducting research, the scholars and educators teaching in graduate programs in communication disorders, and practicing clinicians and their administrators and supervisors.

STUDY EXERCISES

1. Review three of the articles you have already used in previous exercises. Do they provide implications or suggested clinical applications of the findings? What are they? Do they appear appropriate given the findings of the study?

2. Given your personal situation as a student or as a practicing professional, identify and list the barriers to your effective utilization of the research? What might you do to eliminate or reduce some of those barriers?

3. Form a journal club with at least three other class members. Select an article to review and critique. Allow a week for the group to read the article, then meet together to review the study by following the outline in Table 8–1.

SUGGESTED READINGS

Siegel, G. M. (1991–1992). Essential ingredients of a quality MA program in communication disorders: Academic, clinical, research. *Journal of the National Student Speech-Language-Hearing Association, 19,* 84–88.

CHAPTER 9

REPORTING RESULTS OF RESEARCH

MARY H. PANNBACKER

Students and clinicians often are not prepared to write and publish the results of research. What distinguishes the unpublished from the published is a matter of attitude, training, and perseverance. First is a positive attitude of confidence and determination that suggests "I can publish." Second is the probability that those who do not publish do not know how to publish. Throughout their schooling students have had to write, have been graded on writing, but have not been taught how to write for publication. Irwin, Pannbacker, and Kellail (1992) suggest that "university faculty should instruct students about the process of publishing in a journal" (p. 122). Third, an unpublished paper is often one that someone gave up on (Delton, 1985). Fourth, many people think they have good writing skills but few do; good writers edit and re-write — again and again (Henson, 1993).

The purpose of this section is to: (1) identify reasons for reporting the results of research; (2) discuss finding the time to report research; (3) describe the organization and style of research reports; (4) explain how research is reported at professional meetings; (5) classify and describe visual aids, and (6) explain the submission and review of research reports.

REASONS FOR REPORTING THE RESULTS OF RESEARCH

There are several reasons for reporting the results of research including ethical responsibility, institutional quality, professional recognition, improvement of clinical services, and academic survival. Hegde (1994) believes "dissemination of research findings is an ethical responsibility" (p. 442). According to the ASHA Code of Ethics (ASHA, 1990a), "individuals should strive to increase knowledge within the profession and share research with colleagues" (p. 92). In *A History of American Speech and Hearing Association 1925-1958,* Paden (1970) stated, "one of the chief reasons for the existence of a profession or learned society is the sharing of knowledge in the field among its members" (p. 21). ASHA's Committee on Supervision (1985) indicated supervisors should have the "ability to report results of clinical or supervisory research and disseminate it as appropriate (e.g., inservice, conferences, publications)" (p. 60). Defined as research productivity, publication is used to assess program and institutional quality (Bland & Ruffin, 1992; Kraemer & Lyons, 1989; Lash, 1992; Ratusnik, Klor, & Milianti, 1979). Recognition, both individual and institutional, is enhanced by publication (Crane, 1965; Hunter & Kuh, 1987; Lash, 1992).

Research and publication also should be an integral part of the clinical service system (Pannbacker & Middleton, 1991–1992). Ongoing research is necessary to advance knowledge about clinical service and to ensure the provision of quality services to consumers (Connell & McReynolds, 1988; Cornett & Chabon, 1988; Doehring, 1988; Findley & DeLisa, 1990; Hegde, 1994). Furthermore, according to ASHA's (1991b) Code of Ethics individuals should "share research with colleagues" (p. 104). Recently, ASHA's Research and Scientific Affairs Committee (1994) indicated "any suggestion that science and scholarship are not fundamental to clinical practice distorts reality" (p. 22).

Academic survival is related to understanding "publish or perish." Publication has a significant impact on academic survival and other rewards such as promotion, tenure, and merit salary raises (Anderson, 1992; Boice & Jones, 1984; Boyes, et al., 1984; Diamond, 1989; Henson, 1987, 1993; Holcomb & Roush, 1988; Kasten, 1984; Kraemer & Lyons, 1989; Morgan, 1984; Schaefer, 1990). Publishing makes a difference for audiologists and speech-language pathologists employed in a college or university (Burnard, 1992). For example, Batshaw, Plotnick, Petty, Woolf, and Mellits, (1988) found that "those who are promoted have more articles published than those who are not promoted" (p. 741). For these reasons, there is tremendous pressure to publish among academicians (Luey, 1987). Academic survival of students may be related to completing a thesis or dissertation requirement (Chial, 1985; Davis & Parker, 1979; Sternberg, 1981).

FINDING TIME TO REPORT RESEARCH

Most productive researchers have no more free time or no fewer commitments than those who do not do research. Instead, those who do research simply make the time to do it. It is a matter of prioritizing and managing time. Productive researchers frequently have to rearrange both personal and professional priorities to complete projects (Sternberg, 1981). Like anything else, with practice comes efficiency. The traditional approach to writing requires time for warmup and reflection, large blocks of time, and uninterrupted working conditions. Another approach preferred by many involves writing in brief spurts (i.e., writing in brief daily sessions) (Boice, 1989).

Silverman (1993) indicated that research need not be particularly time consuming. Boice (1989) found a relationship between unproductive researchers and maladaptive delays of "busyness" and binging. Busyness involves keeping busy with less important tasks as a way to avoid high priority tasks. Binging is spending most time on a less important activity. Those who are too busy cannot get everything done, whereas bingers are likely to overprepare for classes.

It has been suggested that use of time management strategies might facilitate research productivity, for example, (1) formulating a written plan; (2) generating several ideas for research; (3) identifying times and days that can be scheduled for research; (4) noting times available for analyzing data; and (5) developing a schedule for writing the paper. From the beginning, a target date should be set for completion of the research. A personal deadline should allow for some grace period before the actual deadline. Research must be organized so that it can be completed. If delayed by unavoidable outside influences, it is necessary to work twice as hard the next day or week, or to work over the weekend to stay on schedule (Findley et al., 1989; Kirby, 1989; Kirkpatrick, Rose, & Thiele, 1987; O'Shea, 1986; Schwartz, 1988; Seal & Runyan, 1988; Smith, Carter, & Gilder, 1988; Travers, 1983; Young, 1986). Simply stated, time management is the single most important factor in finalizing the research endeavor.

Related to time management is procrastination or needless delay in beginning or completing a research project. It may include discomfort, anxiety, busyness, or binging (Bernstein & Rozen, 1989; Boice, 1989; Burke & Yuen, 1983; Fiore, 1989; Knaus, 1979). Procrastination may reflect a fear of failure or success. It may also reflect a need to rebel. Carter-Scott (1989) refers to procrastination as the mañana syndrome and describes it as "the precise behavior which keeps you from meeting deadlines, doing what you say you will do, and reinforcing the fact that you are not up to the challenge" (p. 21). Several strategies have been described to reduce procrastination such as cognitive-behavioral orientation, reprogramming negative attitudes, prioritization, contingency management, procrastination support groups, and time slots (Atchity, 1986; Belkin, 1984; Bliss, 1983, 1985; Burke & Yuen, 1983; Deep & Sussman, 1990; Delton, 1985; Fiore, 1989; Fry, 1991; Knaus, 1979). Roth (1989) suggests keeping a research report process log from the beginning to the end of a research project which includes the completed research report (see Figure 9–1). This information also can be helpful in deciding authorship.

In addition, some types of research are less time consuming than others. For example, single-subject research designs require less time to complete because clinicians who use this approach can collect data while providing clinical services (Connell & Thompson, 1986; Hegde, 1994; Kearns, 1986; Kent, 1985; McReynolds & Thompson, 1986; Silverman, 1993). Use of single-subject designs can provide answers to many clinically relevant questions. As Connell and McReynolds (1988) concluded "individual contact with a client over an extended time interval is the basic requirement for implementation of single-subject experimental designs" (p. 1062). This also dispels the myth that there is a division between clinical and research activities.

Date	Time	Entry
Date of the entry	Record time began and ended	Tell what was done. Be detailed and specific.
3/18/94	10:00–11:45 am	Did computer reference search; located articles of interest; requested inter-library for journal articles not available.
3/19/94	1:00–2:30 pm	Reviewed articles.
3/21/94	9:30–11:00 am	Drafted outline and working title.

FIGURE 9–1. Sample Research Report Process Log. (From *The research paper* by A. J. Roth, 1989. Belmont, CA: Wadsworth Publishing Company, with permission. Copyright 1989 Wadsworth Publishing Company.)

WRITTEN REPORTS: ORGANIZATION AND STYLE

English is not written in the same way it is spoken. Competent speakers of English are not always competent writers. Writing is a skill which, like any other skill, must be practiced and reflected upon to be mastered (Ownby, 1987).

The method usually suggested for writing a paper is to first draft a title and an abstract, then prepare tables and figures and finally an outline from which the first draft is written. Most books on research methods in communication disorders contain guidelines for the organization of written reports (Doehring, 1988; Hegde, 1994; Shearer, 1982; Silverman, 1993; Ventry & Schiavetti, 1986).

Research reports follow a standard format that includes a title page, abstract, introduction, methods, results, discussion, acknowledgments, and references. Sometimes the results and discussion sections are combined. Table 9–1 summarizes the information usually provided in each report section. The general form and structure of research reports are fairly consistent across different types of reports such as theses and dissertations, journal articles, and papers for professional meetings (Polit & Hungler, 1991).

In a well-prepared report, ideas must be clearly expressed. Clarity of expression relates to grammatically correct sentences, appropriate word choice, and economy of expression. Several strategies have been designed to improve writing style, including writing from an outline, reviewing published reports, and consulting references on writing style.

TABLE 9-1. Format of an APA-Style Research Report

Title page	Title, name of author(s), and institutional affiliation.
Abstract	Summary of research including method, results, and implications.
Introduction	Not labeled, follows abstract and begins body of paper. Provides logical justification for research to be reported.
Method	Includes sections about method, subjects, apparatus, procedure.
Results	Presents data usually in summary form.
Discussion	Summary of major findings compared to previous research, implications of the research, directives for further research.
References	Bibliography for all sources of information cited.

Source: Adapted from *Publication manual of the American Psychological Association,* 1988. Washington, DC: American Psychological Association, with permission. Copyright 1988 American Psychological Association.

A number of useful guidelines on writing style also have been published (American Psychological Association, 1988; Burnard, 1992; Fiske, 1990; Hegde, 1994; Huth, 1990; Merriam-Webster, 1985; Shaw, 1987; Strunk & White, 1979; University of Chicago, 1982).

APA Writing Style

All publications of the American Speech-Language-Hearing Association (ASHA) follow the style of the American Psychological Association as presented in the *Publication Manual of the American Psychological Association* (1988). A training supplement to the Publication Manual (APA, 1988), *Mastering APA Style* (APA, 1990a, 1990b) is available for students and teachers. Table 9–2 provides a list of journals currently published by ASHA.

Because of its long title, the manual is often simply referred to as the *APA Manual* (Bordens & Abbott, 1988). It provides information about content and organization of manuscripts as well as rules for citing references and arranging a reference list. The *APA Manual* (APA, 1988) also includes guidelines for punctuation, spelling, capitalization, italics, abbreviations, headings, quotations, numbers, tables, and figures.

TABLE 9–2. Journals Published by the American Speech-Language-Hearing Association

Asha
American Journal of Audiology
American Journal of Speech-Language Pathology
Journal of Speech and Hearing Research
Journal of the National Student Speech-Language-Hearing Association
Language, Speech and Hearing Services in the Schools

The seven sections of an APA-style research report were described earlier in Table 9–1. Table 9–3 illustrates some of the more commonly used APA reference formats. All parts of every reference should be checked against the original publication. Furthermore, every reference cited in the text should be listed; conversely, every reference listed should be cited in the text. Mistakes in references are far too common (Day, 1988). Further discussion of inaccurate referencing can be found in the section on Irresponsible Authorship in Chapter 2.

Many journals use APA referencing style. Some journals, however, do not use APA style. For example, *The Cleft Palate-Craniofacial Journal* of the American Cleft Palate Craniofacial Association uses the *Chicago Manual of Style* (University of Chicago, 1982). All graduate programs do not require students to follow APA style for papers, theses, and dissertations. This is unfortunate; students would seem to be better prepared by learning APA style (Shearer, 1982).

Avoiding Jargon and Sexist Language

Vocabulary should be appropriate. Writers should be aware of words preferred by ASHA and those words which should not be used (ASHA, 1992d) (see Table 9–4). Jargon should be avoided, although it is too often used both in speaking and writing. Jargon consists of words that are meaningless and frequently results when words are borrowed from one profession where they have precise meaning and used by another profession (Woodford, 1989b). Academic doublespeak, gobbledygook, bureaucratese, and ostentatious vocabulary sometimes used by self-important professionals and students to impress listeners and readers should be avoided if possible (Barzun & Graff, 1977; Fiske, 1990; Hegde, 1994; Lutz, 1989; Shaw, 1987). Hegde (1991) pointed out that

TABLE 9-3. Commonly Used Reference List Citation Formats of the American Psychological Association

Journal Articles

Stromberg, C. D. (1991-1992). Key legal issues in professional ethics. *National Student Speech-Language-Hearing Association Journal, 19,* 61-72.

Gravel, J. S., & Wallace, I. T. (1992). Listening and language at 4 years of age: Effect of early otitis media. *Journal of Speech and Hearing Research, 35*(3), 58-59.

Campbell, L. R., Brennan, D. G., & Steckol, K. F. (1992). Preservice training to meet the needs of people from diverse cultural backgrounds. *Asha, 34*(12), 29-32.

Book

Middleton, G. F., Pannbacker, M. D., Vekovius, G. T., Sanders, K., & Puett, V. (1992). *Report writing for speech-language pathologists.* Tucson, AZ: Communication Skill Builders.

Book, No Author or Editor

American Psychological Association. (1988). *Publication manual of the American Psychological Association.* Washington, DC: American Psychological Association.

Chapter in an Edited Book

Trost-Cardamone, J. E., & Bernthal, J. E. (1993). Articulation assessment procedures and treatment decisions. In K. T. Moller & C. D. Starr (Eds.), *Cleft palate: Interdisciplinary issues and treatment* (pp. 307-336). Austin, TX: Pro-Ed.

Unpublished Paper Presented at a Meeting

Wynne, M. E., & Grote, M. J. (1992, October). *Reference power through bibliographic data base management.* Paper presented at the meeting of the American Speech-Language-Hearing Association. San Antonio, TX.

Several References by the Same Author in the Same Year

Shewan, C. M. (1990a). Plan to showcase research. *Asha, 27*(1), 62-63.

Shewan, C. M. (1990b). *Task force on research proposal for action by ASHA.* Rockville, MD: American Speech-Language-Hearing Association.

TABLE 9–4. Word Choices Preferred by the American Speech-Language-Hearing Association

Preferred Usage	Avoid
speech-language services hearing treatment	therapy
communication disorder	communicative disorder
client; subject, people	case; patient (except when describing medical treatment)
children with cerebral palsy	cerebral palsied children
person with aphasia	an aphasic
clients with a hearing impairment	clients suffering hearing impairment
children with mental retardation	children afflicted with mental retardation; mentally retarded children
people who stutter	stutterers
subjects with normal development	normals
subjects with normal hearing	normal subjects
speech-language pathologist, clinician, service provider	Speech Pathologist, speech therapist, speech teacher
White, African American, Hispanic	Caucasian, Negro
Down syndrome	Down's syndrome, mongolism

Source: From *ASHA Terminology* by American Speech-Language-Hearing Association, Editorial Services, (1992d). Rockville, MD: American Speech-Language-Hearing Association, with permission.

"long and windy definitions of already obscure terms are a great liability" (p. 10). Huth (1990) believes that pompous slang and jargon can "be seen as coming from an inconsiderate windbag arrogantly wasting a reader's time" (p. 133). Beginning writers may find it helpful to read published research reports as well as consult research references (APA, 1988; Day, 1988; Hegde, 1994), some of which include specific information about word choices.

Sexist language is an error that should be avoided. It is inherently discriminatory language, either spoken or written, that implies an unjustified sexual bias against an individual or a group, usually women, but sometimes men (Schneider & Soto, 1989). Because of the increased awareness that language can perpetrate stereotypes, sexist language should be avoided by speakers and writers (Gefvert, 1985; Kidder & Judd, 1986). Cheney (1983) believes nothing is more pathetic than a writer out of touch with the reality that "women are equal partners with men" (p. 187). One of the most misused personal pronouns is *he,* which is frequently used to refer to someone of unidentified gender such as a child, client, customer, or student (Hegde, 1994; Troyka, 1990; Zinsser, 1988). Indiscriminate use of personal pronouns may imply that all authors, bankers, deans, department heads, doctors, editors, executives, fire fighters, lawyers, police officers, presidents, or professors are male. *Man* is an often inappropriately used noun that also implies sexism. For example, chair*man* of a department or organization. Chair*person,* or simply *chair,* is appropriate. Apparently, there is some truth in Barzun's (1986) statement that "sex is a source of chaos in language generally, as it is in life" (p. 37).

In 1979, the ASHA Committee on Equality of Sexes adopted the American Psychological Association Guidelines for Nonsexist Language (1988). These guidelines provide specific suggestions and examples for gender-free writing. More recently, ASHA (1993b) provided guidelines for gender equality in language usage which include "being specific about gender when inclusion of this information is relevant and avoids generalization which may lead to stereotyping" (p. 42). Other useful references are *The Handbook of Nonsexist Writing* by Miller and Swift (1988), *The Nonsexist Communicator* by Sorrels (1983), and *The Elements of Nonsexist Usage* by Dumond (1990).

Requesting and Obtaining Permission(s)

The legal reasons for seeking appropriate permission when using published materials relate to copyright law (APA, 1988; Day, 1988; Huth, 1990). Most publications are copyrighted; legal ownership is vested in the copyright holder. Permission for reproduction of published material must be obtained from the copyright holder or the writer and publisher are at risk of a suit for copyright infringement of unauthorized use of published materials. When in doubt about the need for permission, it is probably better to request it (Plotnik, 1982). Permission should be sought well in advance. Figure 9–2 is an example of a letter for requesting permission to use a copyrighted material. Examples of letters for requesting permission are also available in Huth's (1990) *How to Write and Publish Papers in the Medical Sciences,* and Luey's (1987) *Handbook for Academic Authors.*

Selecting the Right Journal

Selecting which journal to submit a manuscript to is important. The journals most often used by speech-language pathologists for submitting manuscripts are publications of the American Speech-Language-Hearing Association. These journals are listed in Table 9–2. A number of other journals also publish research related to speech-language pathology or audiology (see Table 6–1). It may be helpful to consult Jackson and Hale's (1990) resource guide for authors which was developed to assist authors in selecting an appropriate journal in communication sciences and disorders for submission.

According to Huth (1990), the following questions should be considered in selecting a journal:

1. Is the topic of the manuscript within the journal's scope?
2. Is the topic represented in the journal frequently or only rarely?
3. Would the journal offer the best match of readers for that topic?
4. What formats are accepted?
5. Does the journal publish an information for authors page or issue similar information that provides answers to these questions?

If undecided about selecting a journal and format, Huth (1990) believes authors can save time by writing or calling the editor and asking for information about appropriate topics and format. Luey (1987), however, says "most journal editors do not welcome query letters" (p. 11). The most appropriate strategy in selecting a journal and format is careful review of the journal's general information, information for authors, and recent issues of the journal.

Rewriting and Revising

Rewriting and revising should not be feared because they are a part of writing (Delton, 1985; Strunk & White, 1979). For most professionals — even those who are prolific writers — writing is hard work. The

Request sent to:

_____

_____

_____

_____

I am preparing a manuscript:

_____

(title of book)

_____

(author/editor of book)

to be published in _____ (approx. date) by

_____

(publisher's name and address)

In it I would like to include the material specified below:

Author:
Title:
Date:
Figure or table number(s):

I request permission to reprint the specified material in this book and in future revisions and editions thereof, for possible licensing and distribution throughout the world in all languages. If you do not control these rights in their entirety, would you please let me know where else to write. Proper acknowledgment of title, author, publisher, city, and copyright date (for journals: author, article title, journal name, volume, first page of article, and year) will be given. If the permission of the author is also required, please supply a current address. For your convenience, you may simply sign the release form below. A copy of this request is enclosed for your files.

Thank you,

Author _____   My return address is: (please print)
      (please print)   _____

Date _____   _____

                                                _____

PERMISSION GRANTED:

_____   _____
Signature   Date

FIGURE 9–2. Request for Permission. (From *A Singular Manual of Textbook Preparation* by M. N. Hegde, 1991. San Diego, CA: Singular Publishing Group, with permission. Copyright 1991 Singular Publishing Group.)

first or rough draft should not be the final draft. Editing and rewriting are the steps to good writing (Dutwin & Diamond, 1991). Most writers go through several drafts (Cash, 1988; Huth, 1990; Meyer & Meyer, 1986). People who compose on computers usually do more revisions as they write than those who write with a typewriter or pen on paper (Roth, 1989).

Most published writers expect to write no less than two drafts of a paper before the final draft. In fact, more experienced writers often continue to see problems that need to be corrected even in the third and fourth drafts. Some writers revise content, structure, and style of a paper at the same time; others revise content and structure first and then style (Cheney, 1983; Hammond, 1989; Huth, 1990; Kurilich & Whitaker, 1988; Venolia, 1987). Huth (1990) developed a series of questions for revising content and structure which are presented in Table 9–5.

Revision, however, should not impede publishability. There is a time to stop revising. Atchity (1986) suggests that a time management decision be made about when to stop revising. After the paper has been revised thoroughly and carefully, the final manuscript is prepared for submission to a journal. Steps in final preparation of a manuscript include:

1. Reviewing manuscript requirements of the journal.
2. Reviewing the final version of the paper to make sure that it contains all necessary elements and that these meet the journal's requirements.
3. Making sure the typed manuscript meets the requirements of the journal to which it is being submitted (Huth, 1990).

After proofreading the typed manuscript and making any necessary corrections, the author writes a cover (submission) letter. Both are then ready for mailing to the journal to which the paper is being submitted (APA, 1988; Huth, 1990; O'Connor & Woodford, 1977). The author always maintains a duplicate copy in case of loss or damage in shipping.

If a term paper, thesis, or dissertation is good, it may be publishable in part (Burnard, 1992; Davis & Parker, 1979; Madsen, 1992). Preliminary surveys, case studies, and methodological or technical innovation or new biographical material—anything that stands on its own—may be appropriate for publication (Luey, 1987). Although the content often is appropriate for publication, it usually needs to be briefer. The format also may require revision although the sequence of information presented in a term paper, thesis, dissertation, or manuscript

TABLE 9–5.   Questions to Ask in Revising Content and Structure of Papers

Title:	Is the title accurate, succinct, and effective?
Abstract:	Does the abstract represent the content of all the main sections of the paper within the length allowed by the journal?
Introduction:	Does the introduction set the stage adequately but concisely for the main question considered, or for the hypothesis tested, in the paper?
	Is that question or hypothesis made clear by the end of the Introduction?
Text:	Is all of the rest of the text in the right sequence?
	Is all of the text really needed or can some be discarded?
	Does any of the text repeat information found elsewhere in the paper?
	Does your first draft have paragraphs that can be dropped?
	Is any needed content missing?
	Do data in the text agree with data in the tables?
	Have you cited unnecessary references?
	Have you omitted references?
	Can you omit any of the tables or illustrations?

Source: From *How to write and publish papers in the medical sciences* by E. J. Huth, 1990. Baltimore: Williams & Wilkins, with permission. Copyright 1990 Edward J. Huth, M.D.

is nearly always the same — introduction, review of the literature, method, results, and discussion (ASHA, 1990c; Shearer, 1982).

PUBLISHING TEXTBOOKS

Scholarly books are issued by five types of publishers: professional associations, trade publishers, university-affiliated centers, university presses, and vanity presses. These publishers differ in their review process, the types of manuscripts they publish, their marketing strategies, and the specific contractual arrangements they make with authors (Luey, 1987).

Some professional associations, including ASHA, publish monograph series. ASHA's first monographs were published in 1954 (Paden, 1970). The Association's most recent monographs, *The Future of Science and Services* and *Proceeding of the ASHA Auditory Superconference,* were published in 1990 and 1992, respectively.

There are two types of trade publishers: (1) general trade publishers who target nonfiction of interest to the general public and (2) specialized or professional publishers who focus on specific professional groups such as the Singular Publishing Group in speech-language pathology and audiology. Frequently, university centers publish books in their specialty areas, although their publications are sometimes limited to research they sponsor. University presses are the primary outlet for book-length scholarly works. They vary greatly in size; some publish hundreds of books a year, others publish fewer than 10. Some university presses publish on nearly every subject; others focus on a few academic areas. Vanity or subsidy publishers charge money to publish; in other words, if the writer pays, the vanity press publishes the book. Obviously, there is no editorial review. For this reason, publication by a vanity press carries no prestige and no merit for tenure.

The primary issue in selecting a publisher is whether the press publishes in speech-language pathology and audiology. A book proposal or a manuscript submitted to a publisher must be in proper form for the publisher. The writer should obtain guidelines for preparing proposals and manuscripts from the publisher to which they plan to submit the manuscript.

University presses and trade houses usually base their publishing decisions on the opinions of reviewers. When a publisher receives a manuscript, it is read by an editor to determine if it is appropriate for the publisher and to assess the quality of the writing. A manuscript may be rejected on the basis of the editor's reading or it may be sent out to reviewers or referees. Publishers often request that reviewers complete questionnaires similar to the form in Table 9–6. A manuscript may be accepted, accepted with revisions, or rejected.

REPORTING RESEARCH AT PROFESSIONAL MEETINGS

Many professional organizations sponsor annual meetings at which research activities are presented, either through traditional oral reports or poster presentations. The American Speech-Language-Hearing Association

TABLE 9–6. Typical Questions for Editorial Reviewers

	Yes	No
Originality and value:		
Is the manuscript a contribution to the field?	☐	☐
Is it original?	☐	☐
Is it important?	☐	☐
Did you learn something from reading it?	☐	☐
Scholarship:		
Is the scholarship sound?	☐	☐
Was the research well planned?	☐	☐
Was it well executed?	☐	☐
Have any major sources been neglected?	☐	☐
Is the documentation adequate?	☐	☐
Are the notes and bibliography in an appropriate, usable format?	☐	☐
Is the information the manuscript provides, to the best of your knowledge, accurate?	☐	☐
Purpose:		
What is the purpose of the book?	☐	☐
How well does the author accomplish this purpose?	☐	☐
Market:		
Is this work important to specialists in the field?	☐	☐
Does it have any value as a textbook?	☐	☐
Will it be of interest to readers outside the immediate field?	☐	☐
Competing works:		
Are there any other books published on this subject?	☐	☐
How does this work compare with them?	☐	☐
What does it add to their coverage of the subject?	☐	☐
Style:		
Is the manuscript clearly written and readable?	☐	☐

TABLE 9–6. *(continued)*

	Yes	No
Is the length appropriate?	☐	☐
Did you find the style appealing?	☐	☐
Organization:		
Is the book well organized?	☐	☐
Is there any repetition?	☐	☐
Is the argument easy to follow?	☐	☐
Special features:		
If the manuscript contains tables, figures, or other illustrations, are they adequate?	☐	☐
Are they necessary?	☐	☐
Are they easy to understand?	☐	☐
Do you have any suggestions for improving the manuscript?	☐	☐
Recommendations:		
Do you recommend that the manuscript be published?	☐	☐
Are extensive revisions needed?	☐	☐

Source: Adapted from *Handbook for Academic Authors* by B. Luey, 1987. New York: Cam-bridge University Press, with permission. Copyright 1987 Cambridge University Press.

holds meetings where speech-language pathologists and audiologists have an opportunity to share their knowledge with others interested in their research. Most state speech-language hearing associations also include research sessions at their annual meetings. Presentation at a professional meeting often is closely linked with publication of the same work in a scholarly journal (Cook, 1989). From an organizational point of view, planning a presentation for a professional conference and preparing a manuscript are identical up to a point. Furthermore, oral reports and poster presentations often precede development of a manuscript to submit for publication.

Presentation of research at a conference has several advantages over journal publication: (1) there is usually less time elapsed between completion of the research project and its dissemination at a professional meeting; (2) there is an opportunity for interaction between the researcher and audience; and (3) researchers can talk with others who are working on the same or similar projects (Polit & Hungler, 1991). On the other hand, oral presentations are not valued as highly as publications in assessing scholarly productivity.

The procedure for submitting a presentation to a conference is somewhat simpler than for submitting a manuscript to a journal. The professional organization sponsoring the meeting usually publishes a "Call for Papers" in its newsletter or journal about 6 to 9 months before the meeting date. The notice indicates instructions and deadlines for submissions. *Asha* publishes a "Call for Papers" section in each February issue. For technical and poster presentations, an abstract of 75 words or less and a summary of 500 words or less are submitted. If the submission is accepted, the researcher is committed to appear at the conference to make the presentation.

Oral Reports

Oral reports usually last between 10 to 20 minutes and frequently involve use of audiovisual aids such as slides, overhead projection transparencies, or printed handouts. They differ from written reports in two main ways: (1) length — usually only a brief amount of time is permitted to report the research, thus the information must be summarized, and (2) style is usually more informal and redundant (Silverman, 1993).

General guidelines for oral reports include preparation and organization. Specific instructions to presenters include: do not "wing it," do not read the paper, and whenever possible use appropriate visual aids to present complex methods and results (APA, 1988; Bordens & Abbott, 1988; Newble & Cannon, 1984). In addition, the skilled presenter: (1) captures the attention of the audience at the very beginning (examples for possible openings are provided in Table 9–7); (2) clearly states the objectives of the research; (3) concentrates on concepts, not confusing details; (4) presents important concepts in several different ways, even at the risk of repetition; (5) uses slides of less complexity than published tables and figures; and (6) prepares for a question and answer period (Cook, 1989; Mulkerne & Mulkerne, 1988; Oliu, Brusaw, & Alred, 1984).

Poster Presentations

Poster presentations have become a widespread feature at scholarly meetings. These presentations are visual displays summarizing recent research on vertical boards and usually require the presence of the author(s) to discuss their work (Simmonds 1984). Unlike oral presentations, poster sessions may last as long as an hour or more (Bordens

TABLE 9–7. Examples of Possible Openings for the Topic Publishing Papers in Speech-Language Pathology and Audiology

Quotation	Almost 80 years ago Place (1916) stated: "Take no reference for granted. Verify the reference that your best friend gives you. Verify the reference that your revered chief gives you. Verify, most of all, the reference that you yourself found and jotted down. To err is human, to verify is necessary" (p. 177).
Narrative	The typical student and professional take the accuracy of references for granted. All too often they fail to verify references. Small wonder there are so many inaccuracies in the published literature.
Rhetorical Question	"Why do so few academicians publish?" Is it that they do not make the time? Is it because they have poor writing skills, or little patience for detail? Or, is it because they are cynical about the editorial process?
Startling Statement	"Many authors are irresponsible. They use inaccurate references and quotations."
Negative Statement	"Improved editorial practices have not eliminated editorial bias."
Comparison or Contrast	"Colleges and universities more often reward speech-language pathologists and audiologists who publish. Public school districts are more apt to reward clinical service."
Reference to Audience's Dominant Interest	"All of you here have a special interest in publishing. Some of you have made important contributions to the speech-language pathology and audiology literature. Others of you are interested in getting published."

(continued)

TABLE 9–7. (continued)

Listing of Specific Instances	"An editor found several inaccurate references in a manuscript, then found many reference inaccuracies in a published article by the same speech-language pathologist. What can this speech-language pathologist do to become more accurate in using references?"
Gradual Narrowing of Broad Statement	"There is limited information in the speech-language pathology and audiology literature about ethical issues of publishing. Publish or perish, fraud and deception, irresponsible authorship, redundant and fragmented publication, plagiarism, and publication bias warrant discussion."
Descriptive Opening	"Ethical issues related to authorship and publication warrant discussion and analysis to ensure responsible publishing practices."
Historical Approach	"Historical reference to irresponsible authorship goes back many decades. In 1916, Place attested to the need for accurate references."

& Abbott, 1988). Several related posters are presented in each session. The purpose of this section is to describe advantages and disadvantages of poster presentations, make suggestions for preparing posters, and identify sources of information about these presentations.

The first reference to poster presentations at meetings of the American Speech-Language-Hearing Association (ASHA) was in the official convention program for 1975 when there were 130 poster sessions. Figure 9–3 presents the annual number of convention papers from 1975 through 1993 classified according to traditional platform presentation or poster session. The number of poster presentations has shown a distinct increase over the 18-year period.

Advantages and Disadvantages of Poster Sessions

The primary advantage of poster presentations is that they permit simultaneous sessions within the same time span (Polit & Hungler, 1991; Yale University School of Medicine, 1987). Poster presentations allow participants to select information of interest, receive substantial information in a short period of time, interact one-on-one with the author(s), and avoid posters dealing with topics of less interest to them (Cooper, Hersch, & Trap, 1988; Polit & Hungler, 1991). They also provide an opportunity for researchers to network with other researchers who have similar interests. For many authors, the poster presentation is less intimidating than a traditional oral presentation (Beal, Lynch, & Moore, 1989). Poster presentations, however, also have disadvantages. First, preparing posters requires more effort and expense than preparing for a traditional platform presentation. Second, posters, like wedding dresses, are often not used subsequently. Third, an author can be seriously disadvantaged by being placed in an awkward, crowded location or may have poor lighting conditions (Simmonds, 1984). It might be best, if possible, to check the room in advance when doing a poster presentation (Deep & Sussman, 1990). Problems brought early to the attention of an organization may be correctable. An example involved placing posters on a crowded stage, which was inaccessible to handicapped participants, while the larger audience area was filled with chairs with no special purpose. Earlier identification and notification might have allowed correction of the problem(s). Fourth, posters are sometimes difficult to transport (Bordens & Abbott, 1988).

Suggestions for Preparing Posters

Those who have been asked to or are considering poster presentations should: (1) obtain written instructions well in advance of preparing the presentation and (2) follow the instructions meticulously (Gustafson,

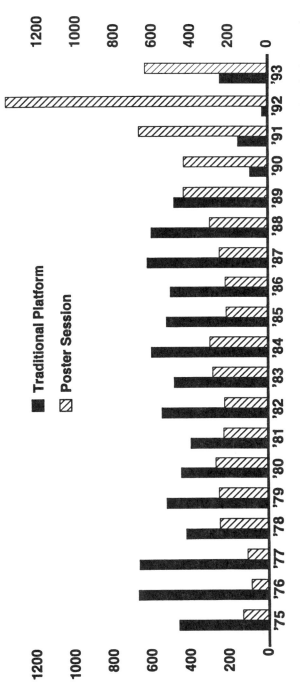

FIGURE 9–3. Number of Papers and Poster Sessions, Presented at ASHA Conventions, 1975–1993, Classified According to Traditional Platform Presentation or Poster Session. (Short courses, videotape conferences, miniseminars, clinical exchanges, and film theaters were not included.)

1981). If the instructions are not comprehensive, the following suggestions may be helpful.

- The text must be readable (at least $\frac{1}{4}$ inch capital letter height) and the line length should not exceed 12 inches.
- Where applicable, use graphs, diagrams, photographs, or illustrations in place of text. Your poster will attract the viewer's attention, and information is more readily assimilated when presented graphically rather than with text alone.
- If possible, figures should be the same width as text paragraphs. This provides for a more attractive format, as well as makes assembly easier and faster.
- Tables are not as effective as graphs, but are more effective than straight text. Key elements or areas on tables can be highlighted, using translucent color film or markers.
- The importance of color cannot be overemphasized. Even a poster that does not lend itself to using figures can be made visually more interesting by mounting text pieces on an attractive colored mat board, leaving 1/2 inch to 1 inch of the color surrounding the text. A double mat, using two contrasting colors is also very effective.
- Take the opportunity to make every figure as visually exciting as possible, utilizing colored film, line tape, and symbols. For contrast, figures can be made with a black background and brightly colored bars or lines.
- Computer-generated color prints are very effective, but can be cost-prohibitive and time-consuming to produce.

Sources of Information About Poster Presentations

Although poster presentations have become a popular method for disseminating research at professional meetings, there is limited information in the speech-language pathology and audiology literature about poster presentations (Beal et al., 1989; Bordens & Abbott, 1988; Cooper et al., 1988; Gustafson, 1981; Lippman & Ponton, 1989; Ryan, 1989; Seaton & McVey, 1983; Simmonds, 1984; Yale University School of Medicine, 1987). Information about poster presentations also has not appeared in the textbooks on research in communication disorders (Hegde, 1994; Shearer, 1982; Ventry & Schiavetti, 1986) except for a 55-word description in Silverman's (1993) *Research Design and Evaluation in Speech-Language Pathology and Audiology.* It may be helpful to review publications about visual presentations such as McBride's (1986)

How to Make Visual Presentations. Some organizations, however, have material available about poster presentations such as ASHA, the American Heart Association, and the Health Sciences Communication Association (6105 Lindell Blvd., St. Louis, MO 63112).

VISUAL AIDS

A visual aid is any illustration used to clarify information in written reports or oral presentations. The most common visual aids are tables and figures. Visual aids are used to increase readers' or listeners' understanding and interest, emphasize significant data, condense information, and integrate data (Lannon, 1979). Simplicity, clarity, and conciseness are just as important in developing and using visual aids as they are in writing (Oliu et al., 1984). Several sources for constructing tables and figures are available (APA, 1988; Day, 1988; Huth, 1990; McBride, 1986; Merriam-Webster, 1985; O'Connor & Woodford, 1977; Paxson, 1988; Plotnik, 1982; Teitelbaum, 1989; University of Chicago, 1982).

Tables are used to simplify information and save space or time by avoiding extended discussion (Hegde, 1991). They usually contain numerical or quantitative data, although they may be non-numerical or qualitative and used to summarize or emphasize descriptive information. Data in figures are arranged in vertical columns with headings. Only horizontal lines should be used to separate data and they should be kept to a minimum. The *APA Manual* includes a checklist for considering tables, which is presented in Table 9–8.

Figure refers to any type of visual aid other than a table such as charts, graphs, diagrams, photographs, or drawings. They are used to convey the qualitative aspects of data such as comparisons, relationships, and structural or pictorial concepts (APA, 1988). Figures should be used only when they provide information that cannot be adequately discussed in the text or presented in a table (Huth, 1990). Preparation of figures is usually more time consuming and more expensive than texts or tables. Furthermore, figures are probably best prepared by professional photographers and graphic artists because of numerous details in format, lettering, and labeling. The *APA Manual* (APA, 1988) provides a checklist for figures which is presented in Table 9–9.

At professional meetings various types of visual aids may be used. These include handouts, slides, overhead transparencies, video tapes, flip charts, and even blackboards. Handouts should be simple in design and easy to understand (Mulkerne & Mulkerne, 1988). They may include a title page with title of the report, author, author's affiliation, and where and when presented as well as an abstract, tables, figures,

TABLE 9–8. American Psychological Association Checklist for Tables

	Yes	No
Is the table necessary?	☐	☐
Is the entire table—including the title and headings—double-spaced?	☐	☐
Are all comparable tables in the manuscript consistent?	☐	☐
Is the title brief but explanatory?	☐	☐
Does every column have a column heading?	☐	☐
Are all abbreviations, underlines, parentheses, and special symbols explained?	☐	☐
Are all probability level values correctly identified, and are asterisks attached to the appropriate table entries?	☐	☐
Are the notes in the following order: general note, specific note, probability level note?	☐	☐
Are all vertical rules eliminated?	☐	☐
Are horizontal rules drawn in pencil only?	☐	☐
Will the table fit across the width of a journal column or page?	☐	☐
If all or part of a copyrighted table is reproduced, do the table notes give full credit to the copyright owner? Is a letter of permission included with the submitted manuscript?	☐	☐
Is the table referred to in text? Does the manuscript include an indication for the printer of the approximate placement in text of each table?	☐	☐

Source: From *Publication manual of the American Psychological Association,* 1988, p. 94. Washington, DC: American Psychological Association, with permission. Copyright 1988 American Psychological Association.

TABLE 9–9. American Psychological Association Checklist for Figures

	Yes	No
Is the figure necessary?	☐	☐
Is the figure simple, clean, and free of extraneous detail?	☐	☐
Are the data plotted accurately?	☐	☐
Is the grid scale correctly proportioned?	☐	☐
Is the lettering large and black enough to read, especially if the figure must be reduced? Is the lettering compatible in size with the rest of the figure? (Freehand or typewritten lettering is not acceptable.)	☐	☐
What will be the effects of reduction on detail and on lettering?	☐	☐
Are parallel figures or equally important figures prepared according to the same scale?	☐	☐
Are terms spelled correctly? Are all abbreviations and symbols explained in a figure legend or figure caption? Are the symbols, abbreviations, and terminology in the figure consistent with those in the figure caption? in other figures? in the text?	☐	☐
Are all figure captions typed on a separate page?	☐	☐
Are the figures numbered consecutively with arabic numerals?	☐	☐
Are all figures mentioned in text?	☐	☐
Is each figure on 8 × 10 in. (20 × 25 cm) glossy print?	☐	☐
Are all figures identified lightly in pencil or nonballpoint pen on the back by figure number and short article title?	☐	☐
Is TOP written on the back of figures to show orientation?	☐	☐
Is written permission enclosed for figures that are being used from another source?	☐	☐

Source: From *Publication manual of the American Psychological Association,* 1988, p. 105. Washington, DC: American Psychological Association, with permission. Copyright 1988 American Psychological Association.

and references. Kroenke (1991) and MacLean (1991) provide additional suggestions about developing handouts. Deep and Sussman (1990) suggest the following when handouts are used: (1) "do not attempt to speak while handouts are being passed out or while people are reading them," and (2) "never pass out a printed handout that does not pertain directly to your talk" (p. 45, 46).

There are several considerations in using slides: (1) slides should be designed specifically for an oral presentation; (2) preparation should be by professionals or at least professional equipment such as lettering devices or press-on letters should be used; (3) lighting in most meeting rooms is less than optimal for slides thus contrast is important; (4) slides should not be too crowded; and (5) slides should be inserted and in proper orientation (Day, 1988). Additional information about slides can be found in Harden (1991), Laidlaw (1987), and Sawyer and Stepnick (1989). Overhead transparencies are also used in reporting information related to research. Factors to be considered in developing transparencies are similar to those associated with slides (Hofland, 1987). In recent years, video tapes have been used to supplement oral presentations. Cost and availability of equipment, however, sometimes preclude the use of video tapes.

SUBMISSION AND REVIEW OF RESEARCH REPORTS

Research reports can be submitted for presentation at professional meetings, publication in a scholarly journal, or both. Often the former precedes the later. ASHA (1990c, 1992c, 1993c) has provided an overview of the publication process and basic information for authors.

Facing Rejection

Rejection and acceptance are central to the research process. Both beginning and established researchers receive rejections, althoughsome erroneously believe that established researchers do not receive rejections and have open-ended acceptance or inside connections (Rosenbaum & Rosenbaum, 1982). Rejection does not have to be final, it should be considered part of the research process (Shillig, 1985). Proposals for papers at professional meetings typically are reviewed by a program committee which either accepts or rejects the proposal. The rejection rate for some professional meetings runs as high as 50 to 60%.

Manuscripts or written research reports are submitted to editors of professional journals for review. The editor's reply will indicate that the manuscript has been accepted or rejected, or that it will be accepted or reconsidered if revised in ways suggested by the editor or reviewers (O'Connor & Woodford, 1977). A request for revision means the topic of the manuscript is appropriate for the journal and that the editor believes the manuscript can make a significant contribution. Editors do not pursue revision of worthless manuscripts. Furthermore, a revised manuscript has $2\frac{1}{2}$ times the likelihood of being accepted (Henson, 1993).

Editorial decisions about what to accept and what to reject are usually based on the following: relevance of the paper to the journal's scope and readers; newness of the manuscript's message; scientific validity of the evidence; usefulness of the manuscript to the journal in maintaining an appropriate range of topics; impact of acceptance on the journal's backlog of previously accepted papers; and quality of the manuscript (Huth, 1990). Very few manuscripts, unless invited or solicited, are accepted unconditionally, that is, without revision (Huth, 1990). There is a basis for thinking that a manuscript will be rejected because scholarly journals are particular about what they accept for publication. The rejection rates in some journals exceed 80% (Irwin, Pannbacker, & Kellail, 1992; Lynch & Chapman, 1980).

If a paper is rejected, the author should consider the reasons given for rejection, and whether the paper should be revised and submitted to another journal. Editors' and reviewers' suggestions should be used to improve the manuscript before resubmission. In other words, authors should consider criticism about a manuscript as an opportunity to improve it (Ogden, 1991; Pannbacker & Middleton, 1991–1992). Furthermore, authors should appreciate "the sacrifice" of anything up to 20 hours of time and (unpaid) effort by reviewers (Woodford, 1989b, p. 112). In recent years, a large percentage of manuscripts, about 60%, submitted to journals of the American Speech-Language-Hearing Association were rejected (ASHA, 1990c). Manuscripts were rejected for the following reasons: inappropriate for the journal to which it was submitted, writing style flaws, not a meaningful contribution, inadequate research design, inadequate sampling, overgeneralization from data, and unanswered research questions (Culatta, 1984; Silverman, 1993).

Although it is uncommon, an author has the option of contesting the editor's decision (ASHA, 1990c; O'Connor & Woodford, 1977). If the author believes the editor's decision was unjustified, appeals can be made to a journal's publication board.

Revision and Resubmission of Written Reports

This is "good news, bad news"—good that the manuscript was accepted but bad that it needs revision. Most manuscripts need to be revised and some manuscripts need to be revised more than once (APA, 1988).

Revisions are accepted by authors as a rite of passage, a necessary evil, and, more importantly, a learning experience. Often, as revisions are made, authors wonder how certain problems identified by editors got by their own careful scrutiny prior to submission.

Acceptances are usually provisional, with final acceptance depending on how well the author revises the paper. It is best to revise the manuscript without delay, and return the revised manuscript to the editor along with a cover letter listing the changes made in response to the editor's and reviewers' suggestions and acknowledgment of the helpfulness of the review. Unfortunately, revisions often are not completed or are delayed. There are no statistics on ABR (All But the Revision), but the number is considerable. The most serious possible consequence of a delay in completing a revision is that the paper will never be published. Prompt completion of revisions is vital to publication. After all, the most difficult part is already completed.

Evaluating and Reviewing Research Reports

Research reports should be read with some skepticism; just because a report has been published does not assure its quality. Published research reports vary tremendously in both quality and value (Ventry & Schiavetti, 1986). Many journal articles are peer reviewed, but in the final analysis, the reader is responsible for making his or her own value judgments about research reports. Bordens and Abbott (1988) suggest a section-by-section analysis for critically reviewing the research literature. The *APA Manual* (APA, 1988) provides a series of questions for evaluating the content and organization of articles. Additional information about reviewing the literature can be found in the section on Consumers of Research in Chapter 2.

SUMMARY

Reasons for reporting research are related to ethical responsibility, quality improvement, recognition, and academic survival. Research is especially important in academia where it has a considerable impact on promotion, tenure, and merit pay. Time management is critical to reporting the results of research. Unreported research often results from failure to make the time to write a report. Various strategies exist to assist researchers in time management. Appendix A provides a list of 131 suggestions and observations on reporting the results of research.

A research project is not complete until the results have been communicated in a report at a professional meeting, a written report, or both. The form and content of oral and written research reports are similar although there are differences in length. The major sections of a research report are the introduction, methods, results, and discussion. Several references on scientific writing style are available such as *The Publication Manual of the American Psychological Association* (APA, 1988).

Journals differ in the procedures used for review of submitted papers and editorial decisions. Manuscripts can be accepted, rejected, or accepted or reconsidered if revised. Very few manuscripts are accepted without revision.

STUDY EXERCISES

1. Select a member of the class or group to lead a discussion of the following questions. The leader should make sure that everyone receives an opportunity to contribute to the discussion.

   a. If it were up to you, would you increase or decrease the importance placed on publishing research? Defend your answer by analyzing the true importance of disseminating research in speech-language pathology and audiology.

   b. If you are a student, are you more interested in teaching, research, or clinical service? In which would you be most likely expected to conduct and publish research?

   c. If you are already working professionally, how necessary is it to do research in your position as a speech-language pathologist or audiologist?

   d. Visualize yourself as the department head of a training program in speech-language pathology and audiology. How would you evaluate the scholarly productivity of the faculty and staff? How much emphasis would you place on their scholarly productivity?

   e. Identify factors in your university or work setting that you think facilitate or inhibit research productivity. How might these factors be reduced or eliminated? (You may wish to include discussion of a reward system, the prestige you believe may be associated with publishing, etc.)

f. Why do you think it is that relatively few speech-language pathologists and audiologists publish?

g. What are the major advantages of publishing? Are some members of the group emphasizing the tangible rewards while others are stressing the enjoyment of inquiring and contributing?

h. Some people are quite knowledgeable about doing research yet remain relatively unproductive. What might be some of the reasons for this?

i. How do people get ideas for research projects? Think of as many sources of research ideas as you can. Everyone in the group should make a complete list of these ideas and continue to add to it.

2. Would you rather submit a paper for publication or present it at a professional meeting? Which probably has more impact professionally? Let's plan a project involving both.

a. You have designed a study on a topic of interest to you in study exercise 18 in Chapter 7. Do you think you would rather present this information as a traditional oral presentation or as a poster session? Photocopy the call for papers forms from the February issue of *Asha*. Read the instructions carefully, then type in the appropriate information and add the summary as though you were submitting your project for consideration. Make sure all forms are filled out completely.

b. Make a handout for participants attending the session. Since you have not actually done the study, list the type of data or information you would include and show how you would format the handout. In other words, do a layout of the handout without including all the specific information.

c. If you were planning to do this session as a poster session, how would you lay out the information on a bulletin board? Use a full sheet of paper and pretend it is the bulletin board. Draw in a design for the presentation with major headings for tables, figures, or photos.

d. If you were planning to do this session as a 10-minute podium presentation, how would your planning differ from preparation for a poster presentation? Make a brief outline of the information you would present along with a list of visual aids and a brief summary of their content.

e. Now that you have laid out a plan for either an oral or poster presentation, which do you think takes more time to prepare? Explain.

f. The same paper has potential for publication. How will the manuscript for publication differ from what you prepared for presentation at a professional meeting?

3. Preparation for publication coincides with selection of the appropriate journal for submission. Name two journals to which you would consider sending manuscripts involving each of the topics listed below. How does an author know if a paper is appropriate for a specific journal? How do scholarly journals differ from other publications?

Phonologic development of children with Down Syndrome
Assessment and treatment of developmental verbal dyspraxia
Language development of children with cleft palate
Risk factors for communication disorders in children
Speech and language skills of children with Fetal Alcohol Syndrome
Speech, language and hearing skills of children with Sickle Cell Anemia
Prevalence of otitis media in low income children along the Texas-Mexico border
The publication of research in speech-language pathology according to gender
Service delivery alternatives for school-aged children who stutter
Effectiveness of an education program to reduce vocal abuse in adults

4. What information would be included in a manuscript for publishing your research described in Exercise 2 above? Develop your answer by following the outline below:

a. What would you include and exclude in the abstract?

b. What are the objectives of the introduction section? What would you include in that section?

c. What would you include in the results and discussion sections? Are they ever combined? When?

d. List and briefly describe the content of the sections of an APA-style manuscript including title page, acknowledgments, references, and so on.

e. How do you conduct a comprehensive search of the literature? Suppose you have the name of an author of an article very relevant to your research. How would you proceed in finding the original article? What sources would you use and why?

5. When an author has completed a manuscript following the format and style for authors of the journal selected for submission, the final step prior to mailing is writing a cover letter. Write a cover letter to the editor of the journal you selected for your manuscript. Make sure you include the title of the article, the author, and a statement confirming that the article is not being considered by another journal or has not been published before.

Answer the following questions about the publication process:

a. What is probably the biggest error(s) in publishing made by most writers?

b. What steps can be taken to increase the chances a research paper will be accepted for publication?

c. Can theses and dissertations be published in journals? How are they adapted for journal publication?

d. Do editors invite manuscripts or do authors just submit them?

e. What do reviewers look for in a manuscript?

f. Describe the sequence of events when a research paper is submitted to a journal for publication.

g. What factors can determine whether a paper gets published or not?

h. What are the chances that a manuscript will be accepted for publication?

i. Hypothetically, if your manuscript is rejected for publication, what will you do?

SUGGESTED READINGS

American Psychological Association. (1988). *Publication manual of the American Psychological Association.* Washington, DC: American Psychological Association.

American Speech-Language-Hearing Association. (1990). *The publication process: A guide for authors.* Rockville, MD: American Speech-Language-Hearing Association.

American Speech-Language-Hearing Association. (1993). Guidelines for gender equality: Language use. *Asha, 35*(Suppl. 10), 42–46.

Day, R. (1988). *How to write and publish a scientific paper.* Phoenix: Onyx Press.

Huth, E. (1990). *How to write and publish papers in the medical sciences.* Baltimore, MD: Williams & Wilkins.

O'Connor, M., & Woodford, F. P. (1977). *Writing scientific papers in English.* New York: Elsevier.

Woodford, F. P. (Ed.). (1989). *Scientific writing for graduate students.* Bethesda, MD: Council of Biology Editors.

C H A P T E R   10

RESEARCH GRANTS

NORMAN J. LASS

- Types of Awards
- The Grant Acquisition Process
- Grant Seeking
- Grant Proposal Writing
- Grant Management
- Summary
- Study Exercises
- Suggested Readings

There is a strong association between research activities and grants. Without grants from the government and private sector, much of the research in communication disorders (and, for that matter, in many fields) would not be possible. For those involved in research, it is essential to locate a specific external source(s) of support for their activities. For example, a university professor or hospital audiologist or school speech-language pathologist who has an interest in a specific communication disorder and wishes to pursue a research project to learn more about the disorder may find that funds are not available within her or his agency to provide the necessary personnel, equipment, materials, travel, and so on that are needed to conduct the research. The only feasible approach for obtaining funds for the research may be through external sources, such as the federal government or private foundations. And the only way to obtain external support is to write a grant proposal to a particular agency. Moreover, the importance of grants is further accentuated in academia, where support of research activities is essential for conducting research, and conducting research is essential for publications in scholarly journals which, in turn, are essential for the awarding of tenure, which is essential for maintaining one's position in a university. Therefore, grants may be the mechanism for job stability and play a major role in the "publish or perish" philosophy in institutions of higher education.

TYPES OF AWARDS

Three types of awards are made for research activities: a grant, a contract, or a cooperative agreement. A **grant** is an award made by a sponsor for a project in which the proposed activity, scope of work, and cost are set by the grantee (an agency outside the funding agency). A **contract** is an agreement to pay for the performance of services that are specified by the grantor (the funding agency). Contracts tend to be more task-specific than grants; however, sometimes the distinction between a grant and a contract is minimal and obscure. In addition, grants are awarded primarily to nonprofit agencies, whereas contracts usually are awarded to profit-making agencies. However, even this distinction is not universal, because some types of contracts (e.g., cost reimbursable) are awarded to nonprofit agencies. A **cooperative agreement** is a mechanism used by federal agencies in lieu of a grant when substantial government involvement is anticipated in the project. For example, the National Institutes of Health (NIH) have intramural programs staffed by their own scientists involved in numerous research projects. However, NIH also has an extensive extramural program involving activities by scientists at other agencies (universities, laboratories, etc.). When the expertise of intramural and extramural scientists is needed for a research project, NIH may award a cooperative agreement instead of a traditional grant.

THE GRANT ACQUISITION PROCESS

Acquiring grant support may appear to the uninitiated as somewhat "mystical" in nature. However, in reality, there is nothing magical about the grants acquisition process. In fact, it is a systematic process which can be considered in three phases: grant seeking, grant proposal writing, and grant management. First the investigator seeks sources of support whose mission and interests coincide with the goals and nature of her or his project. Then she or he writes a grant proposal, following the guidelines established by the sponsoring agency. Then, if a grant is awarded, the investigator manages the research project, including the expenditure of awarded funds.

GRANT SEEKING

Grant seeking involves searching for a source of funding for a specific research project, thus matching the nature of the topic with the objectives of the support source (ASHA, 1989b; Bruskin, 1989; Gelatt, 1988, 1989; Hall, 1988; Polit & Hungler, 1991; Silverman, 1993; Sparks, 1989). There are various sources of external support for research projects, the largest being the Federal Government. Although the actual figure will vary annually because of the variability from year to year in Congressional allocation of funds, the Federal Government awards grants totaling approximately $100 billion each year. In addition to the Federal Government, state and local governments also are potential sources for competitive grants. So are national organizations (e.g., the American Speech-Language-Hearing Association) and private corporations (e.g., Apple Computer Company).

Foundations are another major source of support in the private sector. A foundation is a nongovernment, nonprofit organization with funds and programs managed by its own trustees or directors and established to maintain or aid educational, charitable, or other activities serving the common welfare, primarily through the awarding of grants. There are different types of foundations, but the type that serves as the primary source of support for research projects is the independent foundation. Currently there are approximately 24,000 independent foundations in the United States that award grants. Foundations are carefully regulated by the government and must award grants that total at least 5% of their average market value of assets annually. Although this figure will vary from year to year because of the variability of net assets each year, this requirement translates to approximately $6 billion awarded in grants by independent foundations each year.

Numerous references are available about potential funding sources in both the public and private sector. The following are some representative samples of references available for grant seeking purposes:

1. The *Catalog of Federal Domestic Assistance* (CFDA) is a valuable reference source to learn about relevant federal programs, eligibility requirements, and application deadlines. This information is also available on a computer database, the *Federal Automated Program Retrieval Information System* (FAPRIS).

2. The *Annual Register of Grant Support* is a directory of grant and fellowship programs of foundations, governmental agencies, business, professional, and other organizations.

3. The *Directory of Biomedical and Health Care Grants* includes grant programs of governmental organizations, foundations, corporations, and professional organizations.

4. The *Directory of Research Grants* contains a listing of federal, foundation, and professional association grant programs.

5. The *Foundation Directory* provides brief descriptive listings of private foundations with assets of at least $1 million or annual contributions of at least $500,000.

6. The *Taft Foundation Reporter* provides profiles of 500 foundations that average $4 million in annual grants to nonprofit organizations.

7. The *Taft Corporate Giving Directory* contains information on over 600 corporate foundations or direct giving programs.

8. The *Foundation Grants to Individuals* lists over 1,200 foundations and includes information on scholarships, student loans, fellowships, travel support, internships, and residencies.

9. The *Corporate Foundation Profiles* provides profiles of over 200 of the largest company-sponsored foundations.

10. The *Directory of Operating Grants* profiles private foundations that provide grants to nonprofit agencies for operating expenses (e.g., funds for renting space, overhead expenses, etc.), expenses frequently not provided by most foundations.

11. The *Sponsored Programs Information Network* (SPIN) is a computer database containing information on more than 5,000 federal, nonfederal, and corporate funding opportunities.

12. The *Computer Retrieval of Information on Scientific Projects* (CRISP) database contains information on U.S. Public Health Service-supported research programs.

In addition to the above volumes, several publications provide a synopsis of selected available opportunities to obtain research grants. These include, but are not limited to, the following:

Federal Grants and Contracts Weekly
Health Grants and Contracts Weekly
Foundation Giving Watch
Foundation Grants Alert

Additional information on funding opportunities can be obtained from several sources that publish books, offer workshops, and provide specific information to their clients on grant seeking (and grant proposal writing) opportunities. These include:

The Grantsmanship Center
650 South Spring Street, Suite 507
Los Angeles, CA 90014
1-800-421-9512

The Funding Center
1145 19th Street, N.W., Suite 717
Washington, DC 20006-3701
1-800-852-0001

The Foundation Center
79 Fifth Avenue/16th Street
New York, NY 10003-3050
(212) 620-4230

GRANT PROPOSAL WRITING

Preliminary Considerations

Once the grant-seeking phase has been completed and the agency(ies) located as a potential funding source(s) for the proposed research project, the next major step is to write the grant proposal. However, before the writing begins, there are some preliminary considerations, which follow:

1. Request an application from the sponsoring agency.
2. Carefully review the agency's guidelines (listed in the application material) for the relevant grants program, which should contain the following important information:
   a. suggested format for the proposal
   b. correct standard cover page
   c. any necessary appendixes
   d. number of copies needed by sponsoring agency
   e. deadline dates
   f. any applicable cost-sharing by the applicant agency
   g. allowable indirect cost rates
   h. criteria used to judge each proposal
   i. relative weighting of each factor in criteria.

The guidelines should be followed exactly as specified. If any of the above information is missing from the guidelines, or if there are questions about the guidelines, the sponsoring agency's contact person (whose name, address, and telephone number will be listed in the application material) should be contacted for clarifications.

The Grant Proposal

The grant proposal usually contains the following major sections:

Introduction
Problem Statement (Needs Assessment)
Objectives
Methodology
Budget

Writing a grant proposal is similar to writing a manuscript for publication in a journal or a thesis or dissertation for a master's or doctoral degree, because all include a review of the pertinent literature, a statement of purpose of the research, and a description of the methodology to study a proposed problem. The major difference is that a grant proposal also includes a budget section requesting funds to conduct the research (Catlett, 1989; Kiritz, 1980; Meador, 1986; Ogden, 1991).

Budget

The major categories of the budget usually include the following:

1. *Personnel*—the people who will be working on the project, including the project director (or principal investigator) and other personnel.
2. *Fringe Benefits*—usually includes social security, workmen's compensation, health insurance, unemployment compensation, and retirement plan.
3. *Travel*—funds to travel to professional meetings to present the findings of the research project and, depending on the nature of the research, may include funds to travel to collect data and other related activities.
4. *Equipment*—any necessary instrumentation to conduct the research.
5. *Supplies*—needed supplies and materials.
6. *Contractual*—any necessary contractual agreements with others as part of the research project (e.g., consultants).
7. *Other*—other items not covered in the previous six categories (e.g., telephone and postage expenses).
8. *Total Direct Costs*—the sum of the seven categories listed previously.
9. *Indirect Costs*—expenditures not included directly in any of the seven budget categories listed above, such as the cost of heating/cooling, electricity, maintenance, and security of facilities used for the research project, the processing of paperwork for purchases associated with the project, administrative costs, and other.
10. *Total Project Costs*—the total cost of the research project, including all direct and indirect costs.

It should be noted that grant proposals need not include all seven budget categories listed above. Only budget items that can be justified because they relate directly to the methodology employed should be included in the proposed budget for the research project.

The Idea/Problem

Although following a sponsoring agency's guidelines in writing a grant proposal is crucial for funding consideration, there is still no substitute for the idea/problem being proposed. A good proposal includes a good idea/problem that is expressed well with an appropriate plan for implementation. The idea/problem for a grant proposal should ask a good theoretical or applied question(s) capable of being systematically studied. Some questions to ask (and answer) about the idea/problem for a research study are:

1. Is it consistent with known facts?
2. Is it important (re: discovery, improvement, or application of knowledge)?
3. Is it timely?
4. Is it capable of being investigated (re: the availability of personnel, expertise, techniques, instrumentation, facilities, time duration, etc.)?

Ideas/problems for a research project come from various sources, including the following:

1. the applicant's previous experiences (e.g., teaching, research, clinical practice, administration, etc.);
2. the applicant's readings;
3. unresolved problems in the applicant's field of study;
4. potential applications of previous research findings;
5. sponsoring agencies.

Unsolicited Versus Solicited Proposals

An unsolicited proposal is one that is written without any guidelines provided by a sponsoring agency and is not in response to a particular need or problem expressed by a sponsoring agency. Instead, it originates from a need perceived by the applicant who tries to find a sponsor to support the proposal. Unsolicited proposals have no specific deadline dates for submission and usually are accepted and reviewed by sponsoring agencies at any time rather than at specified dates each year.

Solicited proposals, on the other hand, originate with a sponsoring agency that recognizes a need for something to be done or learned. Solicited proposals usually are announced by a Request for Application (RFA) or Request for Proposal (RFP), which identifies problem areas and sometimes includes specific objectives to be met.

Basic Principles of Grant Proposal Writing

1. The grant proposal should contain clear, concise writing, with definitions for all appropriate terms. (Grants will not be awarded for projects that are not understood by a sponsoring agency's reviewers.)
2. All factual statements should be documented with references cited to support them.
3. An objective and strong case for funding should be presented, with sufficient empirical evidence presented to support the author's position.
4. The idea/problem for funding should be feasible, practical, important, and relevant.
5. The methodology proposed should be well-designed for accomplishing the objectives of the project.
6. The project personnel should be shown (via their vitae) to be qualified to conduct the research.
7. The budget should be realistic, containing only items that are relevant to the proposed project.
8. A knowledge of grant application deficiencies is helpful. The most common deficiencies are: inadequate control of variables; deficiency in methodology; research design problems; poor conceptualization of problem(s); and inappropriate statistical analysis (Thomas & Lawrence, 1990).

Suggestions for Grant Proposal Writing

1. Read the sponsoring agency's guidelines carefully and thoroughly; follow them to the letter.
2. Tailor the proposal to the sponsoring agency's guidelines.
3. Begin writing early, well in advance of the submission deadline.
4. Set deadlines to complete each *section* of the proposal, rather than trying to complete the entire proposal by a certain date.
5. Define a focused problem.
6. Develop procedures to study the problem.
7. Draft the body of the proposal.
8. Develop a realistic budget, with valid justifications for all items in the budget.
9. Add any required additional components to the proposal (e.g., relevant assurance forms regarding the use and protection of

human subjects, compliance with the Civil Rights Act of 1964, and the Drug-Free Workplace Act of 1988, etc.).

10. Submit a draft of the proposal to colleagues for review and comments.
11. Revise the proposal based on colleagues' comments and suggestions then submit the finalized proposal.

Characteristics of a Good Grant Proposal

In summary, a good research proposal, one that should receive serious consideration for funding, will contain the following features:

1. A clearly established need for the proposed research, preferably with supporting data.
2. Clearly stated and sufficiently detailed objectives of the project.
3. A detailed schedule of activities for the project, with clearly delineated and realistic timelines.
4. Commitment of all involved parties verified with letters of commitment in the Appendix.
5. Any relevant cost-sharing included in the proposal.
6. All budget items are justifiable and consistent with the proposed purpose and procedures of the project.
7. All budget explanations/justifications provide an adequate basis for the figures used in the budget section.
8. All major items included in the agency's guidelines are explicitly and carefully addressed in the proposal.
9. All appropriate assurances are properly completed and signed, indicating that all governmental requirements have been followed and fulfilled.
10. All sections of the proposal contain sufficient details and address all relevant issues.
11. All directions in the sponsoring agency's guidelines have been followed to the letter.
12. Appropriate appendixes have been used for providing evidence of careful planning, previous experience, and so forth.
13. The length of the proposal is consistent with the sponsoring agency's guidelines.
14. The qualifications of project personnel are clearly indicated (via resumes, curriculum vitae, etc.) in the proposal.
15. The writing style is clear and concise, thus helping the reader understand the problem addressed in the proposal.

Additional characteristics of good grant proposals are described by Ogden (1991) and Cummings and associates (1988).

The Proposal Review Process

Although the specific process of reviewing grant proposals may vary from agency to agency, there are some commonalities applicable to all reviews. Proposals usually are reviewed by the investigator's peers, colleagues at other institutions or laboratories who are knowledgeable about the topic of the proposal. Sponsoring agencies base their decisions about the awarding of grants on reviewers' comments. Usually reviewers are required to follow specific criteria and use some type of rating scale established by the sponsoring agency to judge the merits of each proposal. Moreover, some agencies, like the National Institutes of Health (NIH), have a very specific rating system for all proposals and a face-to-face meeting of a panel of peers to arrive at decisions for funding proposals.

GRANT MANAGEMENT

Each grant has one principal investigator (or project director) who is solely responsible for all activities and expenditures associated with the grant. Once a grant is awarded, there needs to be competent management of the funds because the grantee is held accountable for all expended funds. In addition, there are reporting requirements, frequently annual reports to the sponsoring agency delineating progress in research activities and fund expenditures. However, some agencies require more than an annual report. The award notification letter or an addendum to the letter should specify all reporting requirements.

Usually funds awarded in a grant are specified and earmarked for particular budget categories (e.g., personnel, equipment, travel, etc.). However, on occasion, because of unexpected expenses or unexpected increases in approved budget items, there is a need to modify the existing approved budget. Most sponsoring agencies have an established rule of allowing the transfer of no more than a specific percentage of the entire budget from specific line items to other specific line items without the need for prior approval from the sponsoring agency. However, in cases that exceed this maximum percentage, the principal investigator/project director must make a written request to transfer funds from one budget category to another and must receive approval in writing from the person at the sponsoring agency who is authorized to do so. The same is true for other necessary nonmonetary changes in the research project: the principal investigator/project director must make a request in writing and must receive approval in writing from the appropriate authorized representative of the sponsoring agency.

Thus, once a grant award is made, the grantee's responsibilities begin. In addition to conducting the proposed research, the principal investigator/project director is responsible for the expending of funds approved by the sponsoring agency (and in the amounts approved) as well as for any fiscal and programmatic reporting requirements. Findley and associates (1990) provide further information about the roles and responsibilities of the principle investigator of a research project.

SUMMARY

Grants are essential for conducting research. The process of grant acquisition is a systematic process that, if followed, should facilitate the acquisition of funds for research projects. This process involves three phases: grant seeking, grant proposal writing, and grant management. Grant seeking is searching for funds from external sources, including governmental agencies, private foundations, corporations, and national organizations. Grant proposal writing involves obtaining a grant application and preparation of a written proposal that makes a strong case for financial support and follows the guidelines established by the sponsoring agency. Grant management involves conducting the research project and expending funds associated with the project as delineated in the grant proposal and approved by the sponsoring agency. In addition, it includes the preparation of fiscal and programmatic reports to the sponsoring agency. Detailed information and suggestions concerning each phase of the grants acquisition process are presented in this chapter.

STUDY EXERCISES

1. Locate and review as many of the following references as possible (most or all should be available at your university in the library, sponsored programs office, and/or department):

    Catalog of Federal Domestic Assistance
    Annual Register of Grant Support
    Directory of Biomedical and Health Care Grants
    Directory of Research Grants

The Foundation Directory
Taft Foundation Reporter
Taft Corporate Giving Directory
Foundation Grants to Individuals
Corporate Foundation Profiles
Directory of Operating Grants
Federal Grants and Contracts Weekly
Health Grants and Contracts Weekly
Foundation Giving Watch
Foundation Grants Alert

2. Prepare a brief summary of one entry (or article) from each of the above references that you read. Include in the summary the following:

   a. title and year/date of reference

   b. title of the entry (or article)

   c. a brief description of the funding program or the contents of the article.

3. Obtain a grant application by writing to an appropriate federal agency (or obtain one from the sponsored programs office at your university). Read it thoroughly and indicate whether or not each of the following items is included in the application:

   a. legislation relevant to federal agency's grants program;

   b. eligibility requirements for grantees;

   c. priorities (topics/areas) for funding for a particular fiscal year;

   d. restrictions (if any) on topics/areas to be funded;

   e. amount of funds available for grant awards for a particular fiscal year;

   f. maximum dollar amount (or range) to be awarded per grant;

   g. cost-sharing requirements (if any);

   h. indirect cost rate restrictions (if any);

   i. cover page and instructions for completion;

j. budget sheets and instructions for completion;

k. assurance forms and instructions for completion;

l. instructions for completion of narrative section of grant application;

m. page limitations for narrative section of grant application;

n. number of copies of grant application needed by federal agency;

o. deadline date(s) for submission of grant application;

p. criteria to be used to judge each proposal, including any relative weighting of each criterion;

q. suggested format (if any) for grant proposal;

r. any necessary appendixes;

s. name, address, and telephone number of contact person.

4. Read two grant proposals that have been funded by governmental agencies and/or foundations (these can be obtained from your department chair and/or your professors) and prepare a brief abstract of each proposal. Include in the abstract the following information:

    a. title of proposal

    b. agency to which submitted

    c. purpose/objectives

    d. methodology

    e. budget summary.

SUGGESTED READINGS

American Speech-Language-Hearing Association. (1989). How to be sure you don't get funded. *Asha, 31,* 76.

Bauer, David G., & Associates (1981). *The how to grants manual: Successful grantseeking techniques for obtaining public and private grants.* Utica, NY: Management & Consulting Services for Not-For-Profit Agencies.

Catlett, C. (1989). Constructing a competitive proposal. *Asha, 31,* 70–72.

Gelatt, J. P. (1989). Obtaining grant funding: Ten steps to success. *Asha, 31,* 67–69.

Hall, M. (1988). *Getting funded: A complete guide to proposal writing.* Portland, OR: Continuing Education Publication.

Kiritz, N. J. (1980). Program planning and proposal writing (Reprint). Los Angeles: The Grantsmanship Center.

Lefferts, R. (1983). *Basic handbook of grants management.* New York: Basic Books.

Margolin, J. B. (1983). *The individual's guide to grants.* New York: Plenum Press.

Meador, R. (1986). *Guidelines for preparing proposals.* Chelsea, MI: Lewis Publishers.

National Institutes of Health. (1989). *Preparing a research grant application to the National Institutes of Health.* Bethesda, MD: National Institutes of Health.

Read, P. E. (1986). *Foundation fundamentals: A guide for grantseekers* (3rd ed.). New York: The Foundation Center.

Sparks, R. D. (1989). Matching ideas and funds. *Asha, 31,* 77, 99.

White, V. (Ed.). (1983). *Grant proposals that succeeded.* New York: Plenum Press.

REFERENCES

Abraham, S. (1993). Differential treatment of phonological disability in children with impaired hearing who were trained orally. *American Journal of Speech-Language Pathology, 2*(3), 23–30.

Adams, M., Aken, J., Bruce, M., Dowling, S., Falek, F., Fox, D., & Waryas, P. (1984). What constitutes excellence in an academic unit. *Asha, 26,* 27–28.

Ainsworth, S., Diedrich, W., Graham, J., Hever, G., Suttan, E., & Hardy, J. (1972). Principles underlying the requirements for the certificate of clinical competence adopted. *Asha, 14,* 139–141.

Alguire, P. C., Massa, M. D., Lienhart, K. W., & Henry, R. C. (1988). A packaged workshop for teachers' critical reading of the medical literature. *Medical Teacher, 10*(1), 85–90.

Allen, M. S., Pettit, J. M., & Sherblom, J. C. (1991). Management of vocal nodules: A regional survey of otolaryngologists and speech-language pathologists. *Journal of Speech and Hearing Research, 34*(2), 229–235.

Allison, P. P., & Stewart, J. A. (1974). Productivity differences among scientists: Evidence for accumulative advantage. *American Sociological Review, 39,* 596–606.

American Psychological Association. (1988). *Publication manual of the American Psychological Association.* Washington, DC: American Psychological Association.

American Psychological Association. (1990a). *Mastering APA style: Student's handbook and learning guide.* Hyattsville, MD: American Psychological Association.

American Psychological Association. (1990b). *Mastering APA style: Instructor's resource guide.* Hyattsville, MD: American Psychological Association.

American Speech-Language-Hearing Association. (1979). Guidelines for nonsexist language in journals of ASHA. *Asha, 21,* 973–1078.

American Speech-Language-Hearing Association. (1984). Software review checklist. *Asha, 26,* 67.

American Speech-Language-Hearing Association, Committee on Supervision. (1985). Minimum qualifications for supervisors and suggested competencies for effective clinical supervision. *Asha, 24*(5), 330–372.

American Speech-Language-Hearing Association. (1989a). *ASHA consumer satisfaction measure.* Rockville, MD: American Speech-Language-Hearing Association.

American Speech-Language-Hearing Association. (1989b). How to be sure you don't get funded. *Asha, 31*(2), 76.

American Speech-Language-Hearing Association. (1989c, April). Final report of the Task Force on Research. *Research Bulletin,* pp. 7–15.

American Speech-Language-Hearing Association. (1989d). The task force on research. *Asha, 26*(9), 41–43.

American Speech-Language-Hearing Association. (1989e). *Plan to showcase research.* Rockville, MD: American Speech-Language-Hearing Association.

American Speech-Language-Hearing Association. (1990a). *Accreditation manual: Professional Standards Board.* Rockville, MD: American Speech-Language-Hearing Association.

American Speech-Language-Hearing Association. (1990b). *Demographic profile of the ASHA membership.* Rockville, MD: American Speech-Language-Hearing Association.

American Speech-Language-Hearing Association. (1990c). *The publication process: A guide for authors.* Rockville, MD: American Speech-Language-Hearing Association.

American Speech-Language-Hearing Association. (1990d). Code of ethics of the American Speech-Language-Hearing Association, *Asha, 32*(3), 91–92.

American Speech-Language-Hearing Association. (1991a). *Annual report: ASHA activities on gender related issues.* Rockville, MD: American Speech-Language-Hearing Association.

American Speech-Language-Hearing Association. (1991b). Code of ethics of the American Speech-Language-Hearing Association, *Asha, 33*(3), 103–104.

American Speech-Language-Hearing Association. (1991c, April). Scientific paper retracted by biologist in response to draft NIH report. *ASHA Research Bulletin,* p. 3.

American Speech-Language-Hearing Association. (1991d). Omnibus survey—Getting in shape: Lean cuisine for the '90s. *Asha, 33*(11), 57–60.

American Speech-Language-Hearing Association. (1991e). Prevention of communication disorders. *Asha, 33*(Suppl. 6), 15–42.

American Speech-Language-Hearing Association. (1992a). *Accreditation manual: Educational Standards Board.* Rockville, MD: American Speech-Language-Hearing Association.

American Speech-Language-Hearing Association. (1992b). Code of ethics: Issues in ethics. *Asha, 34(Suppl. 9),* 1–21.

American Speech-Language-Hearing Association. (1992c). The publication process: A guide for authors. *Journal of the National Student Speech-Language-Hearing Association, 19,* 138–142.

American Speech-Language-Hearing Association. (1992d). *Editorial services, ASHA terminology.* Rockville, MD: American Speech-Language-Hearing Association.

American Speech-Language-Hearing Association. (1992e). ASHA's proposed long range strategic plan 1994–1995. *Asha, 34*(5), 32–36.

American Speech-Language-Hearing Association. (1992f). ASHA's proposed long range strategic plan 1994–1995. *Asha, 34*(11), 35–37.

American Speech-Language-Hearing Association. (1993a). Code of ethics. *Asha, 35*(3), 17–20.

American Speech-Language-Hearing Association. (1993b). Guidelines for gender equality: Language use. *Asha, 35*(Suppl. 10), 42–46.

American Speech-Language-Hearing Association. (1993c). The publication process: A guide for authors. *Asha, 35*(3), 142–144.

American Speech-Language-Hearing Association. (1994). The role of research and the state of research training within communication sciences and disorders. *Asha, 36*(Suppl. 12), 21–23.

American Speech-Language-Hearing Association, Research Division and the Strategic Resources Group. (1991). Getting in shape: Lean cuisine for the '90s. *Asha, 33*(11), 57–60.

Anderson, M. (1992). *Impostors in the temple.* New York: Simon & Schuster.

Angell, M. (1986). Publish or perish a proposal. *Annals of Internal Medicine, 104,* 261–262.

Angell, M., & Relman, A. (1989). Editorial "redundant publication." *New England Journal of Medicine, 230,* 1212–1213.

Aram, D. M., Hack, M., Hawkins, S., Weissman, B. M., & Borowski-Clark, E. (1991). Very low birthweight children and speech and language development. *Journal of Speech and Hearing Research, 34*(5), 1169–1179.

Armson, J., & Kalinowski, J. (1994). Interpreting results of the fluent speech paradigm in stuttering research: Difficulties in separating cause from effect. *Journal of Speech and Hearing Research, 37*(1), 69–82.

Ashmore, L. (1992). Reflections on mentoring. *Communicologist, 17*(1), 9–10.

Atchity, K. (1986). *A writer's time.* New York: W. W. Norton.

Aylward, G. P., & Verhulst, S. J. (1991). Data analysis techniques in behavioral pediatrics: Some practical advice. *Developmental and Behavioral Pediatrics, 12*(6), 370–377.

Aylwin, S. (1988). In search of qualities: Invited comment on Eastwood's qualitative research. *British Journal of Disorders of Communication, 23,* 185–187.

Babbie, E. R. (1973). *Survey research methods.* Belmont, CA: Wadsworth.

Bailar, J. C. (1986). Science, statistics, and deception. *Annals of Internal Medicine, 104,* 259–260.

Bailar, J. C., & Mosteller, F. (1988). Guidelines for statistical reporting in articles for medical journals. *Annals of Internal Medicine, 108,* 266–273.

Bardach, J., & Kelly, K. (1991). Reflections on research. *Cleft Palate-Craniofacial Journal. 28*(2), 130–135.

Barzun, J. (1986). *Writing, editing, and publishing.* Chicago, IL: University of Chicago Press.

Barzun, J., & Graff, H. F. (1977). *The modern researcher.* New York: Harcourt Brace Jovanovich.

Bates, E., Appelbaum, M., & Allaid, L. (1991). Statistical constraints on the use of single cases in neuropsychological research. *Brain and Language, 40,* 295–329.

Bates, E., McDonald, J., MacWhinny, B., & Appelbaum, M. (1991). A maximum likelihood procedure for the analysis of group and individual data in aphasia research. *Brain and Language, 40,* 231–265.

Batshaw, M., Plotnick, L., Petty, B., Woolf, P., & Mellits, D. E. (1988). Academic promoting at a medical school. *New England Journal of Medicine, 318*(12), 741–747.

Bauer, D. G., & Associates. (1981). *The how to grants manual: Successful grantseeking techniques for obtaining public and private grants.* Utica, NY: Management and Consulting Services for Not-for-Profit Agencies.

Baxley, B., & Bowers, L. (1992). Clinical report writing: The perceptions of supervisors and supervisees. *National Student Speech-Language-Hearing Association, 19,* 35–40.

Bayer, A. E., & Smart, J. C. (1991). Career publication patterns and collaboration "styles" in American academic science. *Journal of Higher Education, 62*(6), 613–636.

Beal, J. A., Lynch, M. M., & Moore, P. S. (1989). Views on research: Communicating nursing research: Another look at the use of poster sessions in undergraduate programs. *Nurse Educator, 14,* 8–10.

Bebout, L., & Arthur, B. (1992). Cross-cultural attitudes toward speech disorders. *Journal of Speech and Hearing Research, 35*(1), 45–52.

Bedrosian, J. L., & Willis, T. L. (1987). Effects of treatment on the topic performance of a school age child. *Language, Speech, Hearing Services in Schools, 18*(2), 158–167.

Belkin, G. S. (1984). *Getting published.* New York: John Wiley.

Bell, R. (1984). *You can win at office politics.* New York: Time Books.

Bentley, R. A., Niebuhr, D. P., Gettea, J., & Anderson, C. V. (1993). Longitudinal study of hearing aid effectiveness. I: Objective measures. *Journal of Speech and Hearing Research, 36*(4), 808–819.

Bernhardt, B., & Stoel-Gammon, C. (1994). Nonlinear phonology: Introduction and clinical application. *Journal of Speech and Hearing Research, 37*(1), 123–143.

Bernstein, A., & Rosen, S. (1989). *Dinosaur brains.* New York: John Wiley.

Bennyman-Fink, C. (1989). *The manager's desk. reference.* New York: American Management Association.

Biemer, P. P., Groves, R. M., Lyberg, L. E., Mathiowetz, N. A., & Sudman, S. (1991). *Measurement errors in surveys.* New York: John Wiley.

Bland, C., & Ruffin, M. (1992). Characteristics of a productive research environment: Literature review. *Academic Medicine, 67*(6), 308–396.

Bland, C. J., & Schmitz, C. C. (1986). Characteristics of the successful researcher and implications for faculty development. *Journal of Medical Education, 61,* 23–31.

Blank, J., & McElmurry, B. (1988). Editors of nursing journals: Who are they and how were they chosen? *Nursing Outlook, 36,* 179–181.

Bliss, E. C. (1983). *Doing it now.* New York: Bantam.

Bliss, E. C. (1985). *Getting things done.* New York: Bantam.

Blood, G. W. (1993). Development and assessment of a scale addressing communication needs of patients with laryngectomies. *American Journal of Speech-Language Pathology, 2*(3), 82–90.

Blood, G. W. (1994). Efficacy of a computer—assisted voice treatment protocol. *American Journal of Speech-Language Pathology, 3*(1), 57–66.

Boice, R. (1989). Procrastination, busyness, and bingeing. *Behavioral Research Therapy, 27*(6), 605–611.

Boice, R., & Jones, F. (1984). Why academicians don't write. *Journal of Higher Education, 55,* 567–582.

Bordens, K. S., & Abbott, B. B. (1988). *Research designs and methods.* Mountain View, CA: Mayfield.

Bosshardt, H. G. (1993). Differences between stutterers' and non-stutterers' short-term recall and recognition performance. *Journal of Speech and Hearing Research, 36*(2), 286–293.

Bourgeois, M. S. (1992). Evaluating memory wallets in conversations with persons with dementia. *Journal of Speech and Hearing Research, 35*(6), 1344–1357.

Boyes, W., Happel, J., & Hogan, T. (1984, Spring). Publish or perish: Fact or fiction. *Journal of Economics Education,* pp. 136–141.

Bradburn, N. M., & Sudman, S. (1991). The current status of questionnaire design. In P. P. Bruos, R. M. Graves, L. E. Lyberg, N. A. Matiowetz, & S. Sudman (Eds.), *Measurement errors in surveys* (pp. 29–40). New York: John Wiley.

Braddom, C. (1990). A framework for writing and/or evaluating research papers. *American Journal of Physical Medicine and Rehabilitation, 69,* 333–335.

Braxton, J. (1991). The influence of graduate department quality on the sanctioning of scientific misconduct. *Journal of Higher Education, 62,* 87–108.

Breeding, M. (1992). Mentors and leaders. *Communicologist, 17*(1), 1–3.

Brier, D., & Fulginiti, V. (1990). Duplicate publication and related problems. *American Journal of Diseases of Children, 144,* 1293–1294.

Bruskin, D. M. (1989). Projects of national significance: Assisting members through funded programs. *Asha, 31*(2), 73–76.

Buchner, D. M., & Findley, T. W. (1990). Research in physical medicine and rehabilitation: VIII. Preliminary data analysis. *American Journal of Physical Medicine and Rehabilitation, 69*(3), 154–169.

Burham, J. (1990). The evolution of editorial peer review. *Journal of the American Medical Association, 263,* 1323–1329.

Burke, J. B., & Yuen, L. M. (1983). *Procrastination.* Reading, MA: Addison-Wesley.

Burnard, P. (1992). *Writing for health professionals.* San Diego, CA: Singular Publishing Group.

Butler, K. G. (1992). The meaning of mentoring. *Communicologist, 17*(1), 8–9.

Caelleigh, A. S. (1991). Editorial: Collegiality in scholarly publishing. *Academic Medicine, 66,* 23.

Caelleigh, A. S. (1993). Role of the journal editor in sustaining integrity in research. *Academic Medicine, 68*(9)(Suppl.), 523–532.

Campbell, D. T., & Stanley, J. C. (1963). *Experimental and quasi-experimental designs for research.* Chicago: Rand McNally College Publishing Company.

Cantekin, E., McGuire, T., & Potter, R. (1990). Biomedical information, peer review, and conflict of interest as they influence public health. *Journal of the American Medical Association, 263*(10), 1323–1329.

Carter-Scott, C. (1989). *Negaholics.* New York: Fawcett Crest.

Casby, M. W. (1992). An intervention approach for naming problems in children. *American Journal of Speech-Language Pathology, 1*(3), 35–42.

Cash, P. (1989). *How to develop and write a research paper.* New York: Arco.

Catlett, C. (1989). Constructing a competitive proposal. *Asha, 31,* 70–72.

Catts, H. W. (1993). The relationship between speech-language impairment and reading disabilities. *Journal of Speech and Hearing Research, 36*(5), 948–958.

Chalmers, T., Frank, C., & Reitman, D. (1990). Minimizing the three stages of publication bias. *Journal of the American Medical Association, 263,* 1392–1395.

Cheney, T. (1983). *Getting the words right.* Cincinnati, OH: Writers Digest Books.

Chermak, G. D., & Wagner-Bitz, C. J. (1993). Survey of speech-language pathologists' and audiologists' knowledge of clinical genetics. *Asha, 35*(5), 39–45.

Chial, M. (1985). Scholarship as a process: A task analysis of thesis and dissertation research. *Seminars in Speech and Language, 6,* 35–54.

Clement, C. J., & Wijner, F. (1994). Acquisition of vowel contrasts in Dutch. *Journal of Speech and Hearing Research, 37*(1), 83–89.

Cobb, A. K., & Hagemaster, J. N. (1987). Ten criteria for evaluating qualitative research proposals. *Journal of Nursing Education, 26,* 138–143.

Colditz, G. A., & Emerson, J. D. (1985). The statistical content of published medical research: Some implications for biomedical education. *Medical Education, 19,* 248–255.

Cole, K. N., Mills, P. E., & Kelley, D. (1994). Agreement of assessment profiles used in cognitive referencing. *Language, Speech and Hearing Services in Schools, 25*(1), 25–31.

Cole, S., Cole, J. R., & Simon, G. A. (1981). Chance and consensus in peer review. *Science, 214,* 881–886.

Collins, M., McDonald, R., Stanley, R., Donovan, T., & Boncbrake, C. F. (1993). Severe paradoxical dysphonia. *American Journal of Speech-Language Pathology, 2*(3), 52–55.

Collins, N. W. (1983). *Professional women and their mentors.* Englewood Cliffs, NJ: Prentice-Hall.

Committee on Responsible Conduct of Research. (1989). IOM report of a study on the responsible conduct of research in the health sciences. *Clinical Research, 37,* 179–182.

Coney, P., & Burke, J. (1987). Research and the mission of schools of allied health. *Journal of Allied Health, 16,* 1–5.

Connell, P., & McReynolds, L. (1988). A clinical science approach to treatment. In N. J. Lass, L. McReynolds, J. Northern, & D. Yoder, (Eds.), *Handbook of speech-language pathology and audiology* (pp. 1058–1073). Philadelphia: B. C. Decker.

Connell, P., & Thompson, C. (1986). Flexibility of single subject experimental designs: Using flexibility to design or modify experiments. *Journal of Speech and Hearing Disorders, 51,* 204–214.

Cook, E. B. (1989). Oral presentation of a scientific paper. In F. P. Woodford (Ed.). *Scientific writing for graduate students* (pp. 150–166). Bethesda, MD: Council of Biology Editors, Inc.

Cooper, E. B., Bernthal, J. E., & Creaghead, N. A. (1991). Council of graduate programs 1988–89 national survey: First increase in undergraduate enrollments in 15 years documented. *National Student Speech-Language-Hearing Association Journal, 18,* 126–131.

Cooper, H. (1993). Children and hospitalization: Putting the new reviews in methodological context. *Developmental and Behavioral Pediatrics, 14*(1), 45–49.

Cooper, J. O., Hersch, S., & Trap, J. (1988, Spring). Poster presentations: Technical considerations and format. *Hearsay, 28*–29.

Coren, S., & Hakstian, A. R. (1992). The development and cross-validation of a self-report inventory to assess pure-tone threshold hearing sensitivity. *Journal of Speech and Hearing Research, 35*(4), 921–928.

Cornett, B. S., & Chabon, S. S. (1988). *The clinical practice of speech-language pathology.* Columbus, OH: Merrill.

Coufal, K. L., Steckelberg, A. L., & Vasa, S. F. (1991). Current issues in the training and utilization of paraprofessionals in speech and language programs: A reflection on an eleven state survey. *Language, Speech and Hearing Services in Schools, 22*(2), 52–59.

Coury, D. L. (1991). A guide to critical reading of the literature in behavioral and developmental pediatrics. *Developmental and Behavioral Pediatrics, 12*(6), 351–354.

Cowell, H. (1989). Editorial: Multiple authorship of manuscripts. *Journal of Bone and Joint Surgery, 71*(5), 630–640.

Cox, R. C., & West, W. L. (1986). *Fundamentals of research for health professionals.* Rockville, MD: American Occupational Therapy Foundation, Inc.

Crane, D. (1970). Scientists at major and minor universities: A study of productivity and recognition. *American Sociological Review, 30,* 699–714.

Culatta, R. (1984). Why articles don't get published in Asha. *Asha 26*(3), 25–27.

Cummings, S. R., Strull, W., Nevitt, M. C., & Hulley, S. B. (1988). Planning the measurements in questionnaires. In S. B. Hulley & S. R. Cummings (Eds.), *Designing clinical research* (pp. 42–52). Baltimore: Williams & Wilkins.

Cummings, S. R., Washington, A. E., Irelad, C., & Hulley, S. B. (1988). Writing and funding a research proposal. In S. B. Hulley & S. R. Cummings (Eds.), *Designing clinical research* (pp. 184–197). Baltimore: Williams & Wilkins.

Damico, J. S. (1988). The lack of efficacy in language therapy: A case study. *Language, Speech, Hearing Services in Schools, 19*(1), 51–56.

Damico, J. S., Maxwell, M., & Kovarsky, D. (Eds.). (1990). Ethnographic inquiries into communication sciences and disorders. *Journal of Childhood Communication Disorders, 13*(1), 1–119.

Danforth, W. H., & Schoenhoff, D. M. (1992). Fostering integrity in scientific research. *Academic Medicine, 67*(6), 351–356.

Davenport, H. (1990, Summer). Ghosts who appear by degrees: The strange case of the phantom authors. *The Pharos,* pp. 31–36.

Davis, A. M., & Findley, T. W. (1990). Research in physical medicine and rehabilitation: Information sources. *American Journal of Physical Medicine and Rehabilitation, 69*(5), 266–278.

Davis, C. N., & Harris, T. B. (1992). Teachers' ability to accurately identify disordered voices. *Language, Speech and Hearing Services in Schools, 23*(2), 136–140.

Davis, G. B., & Parker, C. E. (1979). Writing the doctoral dissertation. New York: Barron's Educational Services.

Day, R. (1988). *How to write and publish a scientific paper.* Phoenix: Onyx Press.

De Angelis, C. (1991). Women in medicine. *American Journal of Diseases in Children, 145,* 49–52.

Deep, S., & Sussman, L. (1990). *Smart moves.* Reading, MA: Addison-Wesley.

DeLacey, G., Record, C., & Wade, J. (1985). How accurate are quotations and references in medical journals? *British Medical Journal, 291,* 884–886.

Delton, J. (1985). *The 29 most common writing mistakes and how to avoid them.* Cincinnati, OH: Writer's Digest Books.

Demorest, M. E., & Bernstein, L. E. (1992). Sources of variability in speech reading sentences: A generalizability analysis. *Journal of Speech and Hearing Research, 35*(4), 876–891.

Diamond, J. (1989, July). Publish or perish. *Discover,* 96–101.

Dickersin, K. (1990). The existence of publication bias and risk features for its occurrence. *Journal of the American Medical Association, 263,* 1385–1389.

Dickersin, K., Min, Y., & Meinert, C. (1992). Factors influencing publication of research results. *Journal of the American Medical Association, 267*(3), 374–378.

Dillman, D. (1978). *Mail and telephone surveys: The total design method.* New York: John Wiley.

Dodd, D. K., Boswell, D. L., & Litwin, W. J. (1988). Survey response rate as a function of number of signatures, signature ink color, and postscript on covering letter. *Psychological Reports, 63,* 538.

Doehring, D. G. (1988). *Research strategies in human communication disorders.* Boston, MA: College-Hill Press.

Doms, C. A. (1989, March). A survey of reference accuracy in five national dental journals. *Journal of Dental Research,* pp. 442–444.

Dowling, S. (1993). Supervisory training, objective setting, and grade contingent performance. *Language, Speech and Hearing Services in Schools, 24*(2), 92–99.

Dresser, R. (1993). Sanctions for research misconduct: A legal perspective. *Academic Medicine, 68*(9)(Suppl.), 530–543.

Drew, C. J., & Hardman, M. L. (1985). *Designing and conducting behavioral research.* New York: Peragmon Press.

Dromi, E., Leonard, L. B., & Shleiman, M. (1993). The grammatical morphology of Hebrew-speaking children with specific language impairment: Some competing hypotheses. *Journal of Speech and Hearing Research, 36*(4), 760–771.

Duchan, J. F. (1993). Issues raised by facilitated communication for theorizing and research on autism. *Journal of Speech and Hearing Research, 36*(6), 1108–1119.

Duchan, J. F. (1994). Research to practice: Two approaches to researching child language. *Language, Speech and Hearing Services in Schools, 25*(1), 48–51.

Duggar, D. (1993; January–February). Retractions. Louisiana State University Medical Center–Shreveport–*Library Bulletin,* p.4.

Dumond, V. (1990). *The elements of nonsexist usage.* New York: Prentice-Hall.

Duncan, M. (1992). Mentoring: Even champions have coaches. *Communicologist, 17*(2), 6.

Dunn, S. L., van Kleeck, A., & Rossetti, L. M. (1993). Current roles and continuing needs of speech-language pathologists working in neonatal intensive care units. *American Journal of Speech-Language Pathology, 2*(2), 52–64.

Dutwin, P., & Diamond, H. (1991). *Writing the easy way.* New York: Barron's Education Services.

Dyson, A. T., & Lombardino, L. J. (1989). Phonologic abilities of a preschool child with Prader-Willi syndrome. *Journal of Speech and Hearing Disorders, 54*(1), 44–48.

Eastwood, J. (1988). Qualitative research: An additional research methodology for speech pathology. *British Journal of Disorders of Communications, 23,* 171–181.

Edmonston, N. R. (1982). Management of speech and language impairment in a case of Prader-Willi syndrome. *Language, Speech and Hearing Services in Schools, 13*(4), 241–245.

Eichorn, P., & Yankauer, A. (1987). Do authors check their references? A survey of accuracy of references in three public health journals. *American Journal of Public Health, 77,* 1011–1012.

Elbert, M., Dinnsen, D. A., Swartzlander, P., & Chin, S. B. (1990). Generalization to conversational speech. *Journal of Speech and Hearing Disorders, 55*(4), 694–699.

Ellrodt, A. G. (1993). Introduction of total quality management (TQM) into an internal medicine residency. *Academic Medicine, 68*(11), 818–822.

Evans, J. T., Nadjari, H. I., & Burchell, S. A. (1990). Quotational and reference accuracy in surgical journals: A continuing peer review problem. *Journal of the American Medical Association, 263,* 1353–1354.

Feigal, D., Black, D., Grady, D., Hearst, N., Fox, G., Newman, T. B., & Hulley, S. B. (1988). In S. B. Hulley & S. R. Cummings (Eds.), *Designing clinical research,* (pp. 159–170). Baltimore: Williams & Wilkins.

Feinstein, A. R. (1985). Some ethical issues among editors, reviewers and readers. *Journal of Chronic Disease, 39*(7), 491–493.

Ferketic, M. (1993). Professional practices perspective on efficacy. *Asha, 35*(1), 12.

Fimian, M. J., Lieberman, R. J., & Fastenau, P. S. (1991). Development and validation of an instrument to measure occupational stress in speech-langauge pathologists. *Journal of Speech and Hearing Research, 34*(3), 439–436.

Findley, T. W. (1989). Research in physical medicine and rehabilitation. I: How to ask the question. *American Journal of Physical Medicine and Rehabilitation, 68*(1), 26–31.

Findley, T. W. (1990). Research in physical medicine and rehabilitation. IX: Primary data analysis. *American Journal of Physical Medicine and Rehabilitation, 69*(4), 209–218.

Findley, T. W. (1991). Research in physical medicine and rehabilitation. II: The conceptual review of the literature or how to read more articles than you ever want to see in your entire life. *American Journal of Physical Medicine and Rehabilitation, 70*(1), 517–522.

Findley, T. W., & Daum, M. C. (1989). Research in physical medicine and rehabilitation: The chart review or how to use clinical data for exploratory retrospective studies. *American Journal of Physical Medicine and Rehabilitation, 68*(4), 150–157.

Findley, T. W., Daum, M. C., & Macedo, M. C. (1989). Research in physical medicine and rehabilitation. VI: Research project management. *American Journal of Physical Medicine and Rehabilitation, 68*(6), 288–299.

Findley, T. W., Daum, M. C., & Stineman, M. G. (1990). Research in physical medicine and rehabilitation. VII: The role of the principle investigator. *American Journal of Physical Medicine and Rehabilitation, 69*(1), 39–45.

Findley, T. W., & DeLisa, J. A. (1990). Research in physical medicine and rehabilitation. XI: Research training: Setting the stage for lifelong learning. *American Journal of Physical Medicine and Rehabilitation, 69*(6), 323–329.

Findley, T. W., & Stineman, M. G. (1989). Research in physical medicine and rehabiliation. V: Data entry and early exploratory data analysis. *American Journal of Physical Medicine and Rehabilitation, 68*(5), 240–251.

Fiore, N. A. (1989). *The NOW habit.* Los Angeles, CA: Jeremy P. Tarcher, Inc.

Fiske, R. W. (1990). *Guide to concise writing.* New York: Webster's New World.

Fitch, J. (1986). *Clinical research in communicative disorders.* New York: Academic Press.

Flanagin, J. D., & Newman, R. A. (1991). A profile of clinical coordinators in ESB accredited training programs. *Asha, 31*(1), 67–70.

Folkins, J. W., Gorga, M. P., Luschei, E. S., Vetter, D. K., & Watson, C. S. (1993). The use of non-human animals in speech, language, and hearing research. *Asha, 35*(4), 57–65.

Foreman, M. D., & Kirchoff, K. T. (1987). Accuracy of references in nursing journals. *Research in Nursing and Health, 10,* 177–183.

Fox, M. F., & Faver, C. A. (1984). Independence and cooperation in research. *Journal of Higher Education, 55*(3), 347–359.

Frank, M., & Rickard, K. (1988). Psychology of the scientist: Anxiety about research. *Psychological Reports, 62,* 455–463.

Frattali, C. M. (1990, November). From quality assurance to total quality management. *American Journal of Audiology,* pp. 41–47.

Frattali, C. M. (1991). In pursuit of quality: Evaluating clinical outcome. *National Student Speech-Language-Hearing Association, 18,* 4–16.

Friedman, P. J. (1990). Correcting the literature following fraudulent publication. *Journal of the American Medical Association, 263*(10), 1416–1419.

Friedman, P. J. (1993). Integrity in biomedical research. *Academic Medicine, 68*(9)(Suppl.), S1–S100.

Friel-Patti, S. (1991). A mentorship program. *Communicologist, 16*(4), 3.

Friel-Patti, S. (1992). Reflections on mentoring. *Communicologist, 17*(1), 8.

Friel-Patti, S. (1993). Mid-career mentoring. *Communicologist, 18*(1), 7.

Frohlich, E. D. (1993). Book review: Responsible science. *Academic Medicine, 68*(5), 340–341.

Fry, R. (1991). *Manage your time.* Hawthorne, NJ: The Career Press.

Frye, W. (1991). The origin of the full-time faculty system: Implications for clinical research. *Journal of American Medical Association, 265*(12), 1555–1561.

Gallagher, T. (1990). Asha interviews Tanya M. Gallagher. *Asha, 32*(11), 39–41.

Gardner, M. J., Machin, D., & Campbell, M. J. (1986). Use of checklists in assessing the statistical content of medical studies. *British Medical Journal, 292,* 810–812.

Garfield, E., & Welliams-Dorof, A. (1990). The impact of fraudulent research on the Scientific literature: The Stephen E. Breuing case. *Journal of the American Medical Association, 263,* 1424–1426.

Garrett, T., Bailie, H., & Garrett, R. (1989). *Health care ethics.* Englewood Cliffs, NJ: Prentice-Hall.

Gates, G. (1991). Reviewing the literature. *Archives of Otolaryngology: Head and Neck Surgery, 117,* 168–170.

Gavett, E. (1987). Career development: An issue for the master's degree supervisor. In M. B. Crago & M. Pickering (Eds.), *Supervision in human communication disorders* (pp. 140–134). Boston: College-Hill Press.

Gefvert, C. J. (1985). *The confident writer.* New York: W. W. Norton.

Gelatt, J. P. (1988). The business of grantseeking. *Asha, 30*(9), 43–45.

Gelatt, J. P. (1989). Obtaining grant funding: Ten steps to success. *Asha, 31,* 67–69.

Gelatt, J. P. (1992). Starting a mentoring program. *Asha, 29*(5), 48.

Gerratt, B. R., Kreiman, I., Antonenza-Barroso, N., & Bente, G. S. (1993). Comparing internal and external standards in voice quality judgments. *Journal of Speech and Hearing Research, 36*(1), 14–20.

Gierot, J. A. (1992). The conditions and course of clinically induced phonological change. *Journal of Speech and Hearing Research, 35,* 1049–1063.

Gilliam, R. B., Roussos, C. S., & Anderson, J. L. (1990). Facilitating changes in supervisees' clinical behavior: An experimental investigation of supervisors effectiveness. *Journal of Speech and Hearing Disorders, 55*(4), 729–739.

Girolametto, L., Tannock, R., & Siegel, L. (1993). Consumer-oriented evalaution of interactive language intervention. *American Journal of Speech-Langauge Pathology, 2*(3), 41–51.

Glaser, B. G., & Strauss, A. L. (1967). *The discovery of grounded therapy.* New York: Aldine deGruyter.

Goldstein, H., & Hockenberger, E. H. (1991). Significant progress in child language intervention: An 11-year retrospective. *Research in Developmental Disabilities, 12,* 401–424.

Goldwyn, R. (1987). Manuscript acceptance: Excellence not favoritism. *Plastic and Reconstructive Surgery, 74,* 827–828.

Goldwyn, R. (1990). Scheming not writing for publication. *Plastic and Reconstructive Surgery, 77,* 281–282.

Gow, M. L., & Ingham, R. J. (1992). Modifying electrographic identified intervals of phonation: The effect on stuttering. *Journal of Speech and Hearing Research, 35*(3), 495–511.

Groves, R. M. (1989). *Survey errors and survey costs.* New York: John Wiley.

Groves, R. M., Biener, P. B., Lyberg, L. E., Massey, J. T., Nicholls, W. L., & Waksbug, J. (1989). *Telephone survey methodology.* New York: John Wiley.

Guitar, B., Kopff Schaefer, H., Donahue-Kilburg, G., & Bond, L. (1992). Parent verbal interactions and speech rate: A case study in stuttering. *Journal of Speech and Hearing Research, 35*(4), 742–754.

Gustafson, M. (1981). Poster presentation more than a poster on a board. *Journal of Continuing Education in Nursing, 12*(1), 28–30.

Gutierrez-Clellen, V. P., & Heinrichs-Ramos, L. H. (1993). Cohesion in the narrative of Spanish-speaking children: A developmental study. *Journal of Speech and Hearing Research, 36*(3), 559–567.

Hall, M. (1988). *Getting funded: A complete guide to proposal writing.* Portland, OR: Continuing Education Publications.

Hall, N. E., Yamashita, T. S., & Aran, D. M. (1993). Relationship between language and fluency in children with developmental language disorders. *Journal of Speech and Hearing Research, 36*(3), 568–579.

Halls, S., Larrigan, L. B., & Madison, C. L. (1991). A comparison of speech-language pathologists in rural and urban school districts in the state of Washington. *Language, Speech and Hearing Services in Schools, 22*(4), 204–210.

Hambrecht, G., & Sarris, T. L. (1993). Self-supervision training with beginning clinicians. *National Student Speech-Language-Hearing Association Journal, 20,* 60–64.

Hammond, E. (1989). *Critical thinking, thoughtful writing.* New York: McGraw-Hill.

Harden, R. M. (1991). Twelve tips on using double slide projection. *Asha, 13*(4), 267–271.

Hargrove, P. M. (1982). Misarticulated vowels: A case study. *Language, Speech and Hearing Services in Schools, 13*(2), 86–95.

Harrison, T., Silman, S., & Silverman, C. A. (1989). Contralateral acoustic-reflex growth function in a patient with a cerebellar tumor: A case study. *Journal of Speech and Hearing Disorders, 54*(4), 505–509.

Hartman, D. E., Daily, W. W., & Morin, K. N. (1989). A case of superior laryngeal nerve paresis and psychogenic dysphonia. *Journal of Speech and Hearing Disorders, 54*(4), 526–529.

Hearst, N., & Hulley, S. B. (1988). Using secondary data. In S. B. Hulley & S. R. Cummings (Eds.), *Designing clinical research* (pp. 53–62). Baltimore: Williams & Wilkins.

Hegde, M. N. (1991). *Singular manual of textbook preparation.* San Diego, CA: Singular Publishing Group.

Hegde, M. N. (1994). *Clinical research in communicative disorders.* Austin, TX: Pro-Ed.

Henri, B. P. (1994). Graduate student preparation: Tomorrow's challenge. *Asha, 36*(1), 43–46.

Henson, K. T. (1986, April). Writing for publication: Play to win. *Phi Delta Kappan,* pp. 602–604.

Henson, K. T. (1987, December). Writing for professional publication. *Phi Delta Kappan,* pp. 800–803.

Henson, K. T. (1990, June). Writing for education journals. *Phi Delta Kappan,* pp. 800–803.

Henson, K. T. (1993, June). Writing for successful publication: Advice from editors. *Phi Delta Kappan,* pp. 799–802.

Herrington-Hall, B. L., Lee, L., Stemple, J. C., Niemi, K. R., & McHune, M. M. (1988). Description of laryngeal pathologies by age, sex, and occupation in a treatment-seeking sample. *Journal of Speech and Hearing Disorders, 53*(1), 57–64.

Hillis, J. W. (1993). Ongoing assessment in the management of stuttering: A clinical perspective. *American Journal of Speech-Language Pathology, 2*(1), 24–36.

Hoaglin, D. C., Mosteller, F., & Tukey, J. W. (1991). *Fundamentals of exploratory analysis of variance.* New York: John Wiley.

Hockelman, R. A. (1992). A pediatrician's view: Editorial ethics. *Pediatric Annals, 21*(5), 277–278.

Hoffman, P. R., Norris, T. A., & Monjure, J. (1990). Comparison of process targeting and whole language treatments for phonologically delayed preschool children. *Language, Speech and Hearing Services in Schools, 21*(2), 102–109.

Hofland, S. L. (1987). Transparency design for effective oral presentations. *Journal of Continuing Education in Nursing, 18*(3), 83–88.

Holcomb, J., & Roush, R. (1988). A study of the scholarly activities of allied health facilities in southern academic health science centers. *Journal of Allied Health, 17*(11), 277–293.

Holzemer, W. L. (1988). Academic fraud. *Journal of Nursing Education, 27,* 309.

Horowitz, L. (1988). *Knowing where to look: The ultimate guide to research.* Cincinnati, OH: Writer's Digest Books.

Huck, S. W., Cormier, W. H., & Bounds, W. G. (1974). *Reading statistics and research.* New York: HarperCollins.

Hunter, A., & Kuh, G. (1987). The "white wing." Journal of Higher Education, *58*(4), 443–462.

Huth, E. J. (1986). Irresponsible authorship and wasteful publication. *Annals of Internal Medicine, 104,* 257–258.

Huth, E. J. (1990). *How to write and publish papers in the medical sciences.* Baltimore: Williams & Wilkins.

Hux, K., Morris-Friche, M., & Sanger, D. D. (1993). Language sampling practices: A survey of nine states. *Language, Speech and Hearing Services in Schools, 24*(2), 84–91.

Irby, D. M. (1993). Faculty development and academic vitality. *Academic Medicine, 68*(10), 760–763.

Ingham, R. J., Cordes, A. K., & Finn, P. (1993). Time-interval measurement of stuttering: Systematic replication of Ingham, Cordes, and Gow (1993). *Journal of Speech and Hearing Research, 36*(6), 1168–1176.

Irwin, D. L., Pannbacker, M. D., & Kellail, K. (1992). Writing for publication in communication disorders and related journals. *Journal of the National Student Speech-Language-Hearing Association, 19,* 119–122.

Isaac, S., & Michael, W. B. (1987). *Handbook in research and evaluation.* San Diego: Edits Publishers.

Jackson, P., & Hale, S. (1990). *Journals in communication sciences and disorders: A resource guide for authors.* Rockville, MD: American Speech-Language-Hearing Association.

Jenuchim, J., & Shapiro, P. (1992). *Women, mentors, and success.* New York: Fawcett Columbia.

Johnson, C. E., Stein, R. I., & Lass, N. J. (1992). Public school nurses: A preparedness for a hearing aid monitoring program. *Language, Speech and Hearing Services in Schools, 23*(2), 141–144.

Johnson, S. B. (1991). Methodological considerations in pediatric behavioral research: Measurements. *Developmental and Behavioral Pediatrics, 12*(6), 361–369.

Johnston, M. V., Findley, T. W., DeLuca, J., & Katz, R. T. (1991). Research in physical medicine and rehabilitation. XII: Measurement tools with application to brain injury. *American Journal of Physical Medicine and Rehabilitation, 70*(1), 40–56.

Jowers, L. T., & Herr, L. (1990). A review of literature on mentor-protege relationships. In G. Clayton & P. Baj (Eds.), *Review of research in nursing education* (pp. 49–77). New York: New York League for Nursing.

Kalichman, M. W., & Friedman, P. J. (1992). A pilot study of biomedical trainees' perceptions concerning research ethics. *Academic Medicine, 67*(11), 769–775.

Kamhi, A. G. (1984). Problem solving in child language disorders: The clinical scientist. *Language, Speech and Hearing Services in Schools, 15*, 226–234.

Kamhi, A. G. (1993). Research into practice: Some problems with the marriage between theory and practice. *Language, Speech and Hearing Services in Schools, 24*(1), 57–60.

Kamhi, A. G. (1994a). Research into practice: Introduction. *Language, Speech and Hearing Services in Schools, 25*(1), 471.

Kamhi, A. G. (1994b). Research into practice: Toward a theory of clinical expertise in speech-language pathology. *Language, Speech and Hearing Services in Schools, 24*(2), 115–118.

Kasten, K. (1984). Tenure and merit pay as rewards for research, teaching, service at a research university. *Journal of Higher Education, 55*, 500–514.

Kearns, K. (1986). Flexibility of single-subject experimental designs: Design selection and arrangement of experimental phases. *Journal of Speech and Hearing Disorders, 51*, 204–214.

Kent, R. D. (1983). Role of research. *Procedures of the 1983 National Conference on Undergraduate, Graduate and Continuing Education* (ASHA Reports No. 13) 76–86. Rockville, MD: American Speech-Language-Hearing Association.

Kent, R. D. (1985). Science and the clinician: The practice of science and the science of practice. *Seminars in Speech and Language, 6*, 1–12.

Kent, R. D. (1989–1990). Fragmentation of clinical service and clinical science in communication disorders. *National Student Speech-Language-Hearing Association Journal, 17*, 4–16.

Kent, R. D., Sufit, R. L., Rosenbek, J. C., Kent, J. F., Weisman, G., Martin, R. E., & Brooks, B. R. (1991). Speech deterioration in amyotrophic lateral sclerosis: A case study. *Journal of Speech and Hearing Research, 34*(6), 1269–1275.

Keough, K. (1990). Emerging issues for the profession in the 1990s. *Asha, 32*(8), 55–60.

Kerlinger, F. N. (1973). *Foundations of behavioral research.* New York: Holt, Rinehart & Winston.

Kidder, I., & Judd, C. (1986). *Research methods in social relations.* New York: Holt, Rinehart & Winston.

Kirby, R. (1989). Excellence in rehabilitation through research. *American Journal of Physical Medicine and Rehabilitation, 68,* 43–44.

Kiritz, N. J. (1980). *Program planning and proposal writing.* Los Angeles: The Grantsmanship Center.

Kirpatrick, M., Rose, M., & Thiele, R. (1987). Faculty workload measures: The time is right. *Journal of Nursing Education, 26,* 84–86.

Kirsling, R. A., & Kochar, M. S. (1990). Mentors in graduate medical education at the Medical College of Wisconsin. *Academic Medicine, 65,* 272–274.

Klein, D. F. (1993). Should the government assure scientific integrity? *Academic Medicine, 68*(9) (Suppl.), 56–59.

Knaus, W. J. (1979). *Do it now: How to stop procrastinating.* Englewood Cliffs, NJ: Prentice-Hall.

Koppel, G. (1993). *Design and analysis: A researcher's handbook.* Englewood Cliffs, NJ: Prentice-Hall.

Korenman, S. G. (1993). Conflicts of interest and commercialization of research. *Academic Medicine, 68*(9)(Suppl.), 18–22.

Kornblut, A. (1988). Some thoughts on writing a paper for publication. *ENT Journal, 67,* 711–712.

Kovach, T. M., & Moore, M. S. (1992). Leaders are born through the mentoring process. *Asha, 29*(1), 33–35, 47.

Kovarsky, D., & Crago, M. (1991). Toward the ethnography of communication disorders. *National Student Speech-Language-Hearing Association Journal, 18,* 44–55.

Kraemer, G., & Lyons, K. (1989, Spring). Research productivity of allied health faculty in academic health centers. *Journal of Allied Health, 18,* pp. 349–359.

Krathwohl, D. (1985). *Social and behavioral science research.* San Francisco, CA: Jossey-Bass.

Kreiman, J., Gerratt, B. R., Kempston, G. B., Erman, A., & Berker, G. S. (1993). Perceptual evaluation of voice quality: Review, tutorial, and a framework for future research. *Journal of Speech and Hearing Research, 36*(1), 21–40.

Kroenke, K. (1991). Handouts: Making the lecture portable. *Medical Teacher, 13*(3), 199–203.

Krogh, C. L. (1985). A checklist system for critical review of medical literature. *Medical Education, 19,* 392–395.

Kurilich, F., & Whitaker, H. (1988). *Writing strategy for student writers.* New York: Holt, Rinehart & Winston.

Kuzma, J. W. (1984). *Basic statistics for the health sciences.* Mountain View, CA: Mayfield.

Kwiatkowski, J., & Shriberg, L. D. (1993). Speech normalization in developmental phonological disorders: A retrospective study of capability-focus theory. *Language, Speech and Hearing Services in Schools, 24*(1), 10–18.

Laidlaw, J. M. (1987). Twelve tape-slide tips: Some helpful hints for the producers of tape/slide material. *Medical Teacher, 9*(2), 139–144.

Lankford, J. E., & West, D. M. (1993). A study of noise exposure and hearing sensitivity in a high school wood working class. *Language, Speech and Hearing Services in Schools, 24*(3), 167–173.

Lanks, K. W. (1990). *Academic environment.* Brooklyn Faculty Press.

Lannon, J. M. (1979). *Technical writing.* Boston: Little, Brown.

Lash, A. A. (1992). Determinants of career attainments of doctorates in nursing. *Nursing Research, 41*(4), 216–222.

Lass, N. J., Middleton, G. F., Pannbacker, M. D., & Marks, C. J. (1993). A survey of speech-language pathologists' career development and satisfaction. *National Student Speech-Language-Hearing Association Journal, 20,* 99–104.

Lass, N. J., Ruscello, D. M., Schmidt, J. F., Pannbacker, M. D., Orlando, M. B., Dean, K. A., Ruziska, J. C., & Bradshaw, K. H. (1992). Teachers' perceptions of stutters. *Language, Speech and Hearing Services in Schools, 23*(1), 78–81.

Lass, N. J., Woodford, C. M., & Everly-Myers, D. S. (1990). A survey of college students' knowledge and awareness of hearing, hearing loss, and hearing health. *National Student Speech-Language-Hearing Association Journal, 17,* 90–95.

Leedy, P. D. (1989). *Practical research.* New York: Macmillan.

Lefferts, R. (1983). *Basic handbook of grants management.* New York: Basic Books.

Lieske, A. M. (1986). *Clinical nursing research: A guide to undertaking and using research in nursing practice.* Rockville, MD: Aspen Publications.

Light, J., Dattilo, J., English, J., Gutierrez, R., & Hartz, J. (1992). Instructing facilitators to support the communication of people who use augmentative systems. *Journal of Speech and Hearing Research, 35*(4), 865–875.

Lippman, D. T., & Ponton, K. S. (1989). Designing a research poster with impact. *Western Journal of Nursing Research, 11,* 477–485.

Lo, B., Feigal, D., Cummings, S. R., & Hulley, S. B. (1988). Addressing ethical issues. In S. B. Hulley, & S. R. Cummings (Eds.), *Designing clinical research* (pp. 151–158). Baltimore: Williams & Wilkins.

Loflaud, J., & Loflaud, L. H. (1984). *Analyzing social settings: A guide to qualitative observation and analysis.* Belmont, CA: Wadsworth.

Loftin, B. P. (1987). Learning from role models and mentors. In R. Bard, C. Bell, L. Stephen, & L. Webster (Eds.), *The trainer's professional development handbook* (pp. 71–80). San Francisco: Jossey-Bass.

Ludlow, C. L. (1986). The research career ladder in human communication sciences and disorders. In R. M. McLauchlin (Ed.), *Speech-language pathology and audiology: Issues and management* (pp. 409–424). New York: Grune & Stratton.

Luey, B. (1987). *Handbook for academic authors.* New York: Cambridge University Press.

Lundberg, G. D., & Williams, E. (1991). The quality of a medical article. *Journal of the American Medical Association, 265,* 1161–1162.

Lutz, W. (1989). *Double-speak.* New York: Harper & Row.

Lynch, B., & Chapman, C., (1980). *Writing for communication in science and medicine.* New York: Van Nostrand Reinhold.

MacLean, I. (1991). Twelve tips on providing handouts. *Medical Teacher, 13*(1), 7–12.

Madsen, D. (1992). *Successful dissertations and theses.* San Francisco, CA: Jossey-Bass.

Mahr, G., & Leith, W. (1992). Psychogenic stuttering of adult onset. *Journal of Speech and Hearing Research, 35*(2), 283–286.

Malinoff, R., & Spivak, L. G. (1991). The professional doctorate. *Asha, 31*(9), 51–54.

Manifold, J. A. Y., & Murdoch, B. E. (1993). Speech breathing in young adults: Effect of body type. *Journal of Speech and Hearing Research, 36*(4), 657–671.

Mansour, S. L., & Punch, J. L. (1984). Research activity among ASHA members. *Asha, 26*(12), 41–42.

Margolin, J. B. (1983). *The individual's guide to grants.* New York: Plenum Press.

Maxfield, M., Schweitzer, J., & Gouvier, W. D. (1988). Measures of central tendency, variability, and relative standing in non-normal distributions: Alternatives to the mean and standard score. *Archives of Physical Medicine Rehabilitation, 69,* 406–409.

McAleer, S. (1990). Twelve tips for using statistics. *Medical Teacher, 12(2),* 127–130.

McBride, D. (1986). *How to make visual presentations.* New York: Art Direction Book Company.

McCall, G. J., & Simmons, J. L. (1969). *Issues in participant observation.* New York: Random House.

McFarlane, L. A., & Hagler, P. (1993). Teams and teamwork: Academic settings. *Asha, 30*(7), 37–38, 48.

McHalffey, P. B., & Pannbacker, M. (1992). Perceived sources and level of stress in speech-language pathology students. *National Student Speech-Language-Hearing Association Journal, 19,* 123–127.

McReynolds, L. V., & Thompson, C. K. (1986). Flexibility of single subject experimental designs. Part II: Review of the basics of single subject designs. *Journal of Speech and Hearing Disorders, 51,* 194–203.

Meador, R. (1986). *Guidelines for preparing proposals.* Chelsea, MI: Lewis Publishers.

Medsen, D. (1992). *Successful dissertations and theses.* San Francisco: Jossey-Bass.

Merriam-Webster. (1985). *Webster's standard American style manual,* Springfield, MA: Merriam-Webster.

Metz, D. E., & Folkins, J. W. (1985). Protection of human subjects in speech and hearing research. *Asha, 27*(3), 25–29.

Meyer, H. E., & Meyer, J. M. (1986). *How to write.* Washington, DC: Storm King Press.

Micheli, S. (1992). The name of the game is . . . documentation. *Hearsay, 7*(1), 22–28.

Middleton, G. F., & Pannbacker, M. H. (1992). Gender differences in research productivity: Asha publications 1960–1991.

Miller, C., & Swift, K. (1988). *The handbook of nonsexist writing.* New York: Harper & Row.

Miller, R. (1987). *Evaluating faculty for promotion and tenure.* San Francisco, CA: Jossey-Bass.

Miller, S. Q., Miller, J. K., & Madison, C. L. (1980). A speech and language clinician's involvement in a PL-142 public hearing: A case study. *Language, Speech and Hearing Services in Schools, 11*(2), 75–84.

Mineo, B. A., & Goldstein, H. (1990). Generalized learning of receptive and expressive action-object responses by language delayed preschoolers. *Journal of Speech and Hearing Disorders, 55*(4), 665–678.

Moll, K. (1983). Graduate education. *Proceedings of the 1983 National Conference on Undergraduate, Graduate, and Continuing Education* (ASHA Reports No. 13), pp. 25–37.

Monahan, D. (1986). Remediation of common phonological processes: Four case studies. *Language, Speech and Hearing Services in Schools, 17*(3), 199–206.

Montgomery, J. W. (1993). Haptic recognition in children with specific language impairment: Effects of response modality. *Journal of Speech and Hearing Research, 36*(1), 98–104.

Moore, K. (1982). The role of mentors in developing leaders for academia. *Educational Record, 63,* 23–28.

Moran, M. J. (1993). Final consonant deletion in African American children speaking Black English: A closer look. *Language, Speech and Hearing Services in Schools, 24*(3), 161–166.

Morgan, P. (1984, January 15). Journal publication and academic careers: Publish or perish. *Canadian Medical Association Journal, 130,* p. 96.

Morrow, D. R., Mirendo, P., Berkelman, D. R., & Yorkston, K. M. (1993). Vocabulary selection for augmentative communication systems: A comparison of three techniques. *American Journal of Speech-Language Pathology, 2*(2), 19–30.

Mulkerne, D. J. D., & Mulkerne, D. J. D. (1988). *The perfect term paper: Step by step.* New York: Doubleday.

Muma, J. R. (1993). The need for replication. *Journal of Speech and Hearing Research, 36*(5), 927–930.

Nass, J. F., & Flahire, M. J. (1991). Preprofessional only program: A fruitful endeavor. *Asha, 28*(1), 39–41.

National Institutes of Health. (1989). *Preparing a research grant application to the National Institutes of Health.* Bethesda, MD: National Institutes of Health.

Neeley, R. A., McDaniel, D. M., & Perez, E. (1991). NSSLHA survey. *National Student Speech-Language-Hearing Association Journal, 18,* 132–136.

Nemko, M. (1988). *How to have an Ivy League experience at state universities.* New York: Avon.

Neumann, Y., & Finaly-Neuhaus, E. (1991). The support-stress paradigm and faculty research publications. *Journal of Higher Education, 61,* 565–580.

Newble, D. I., & Cannon, R. A. (1984). How to make a presentation at a scientific meeting. *Medical Teacher, 6*(1), 6–9.

Norman, K. (1986). Importance of factors in the review of grant proposals. *Journal of Applied Psychology, 71*(1), 156–182.

Northern, J. L. (1989). *Study guide for handbook of speech-language pathology and audiology.* Philadelphia: B. C. Decker.

O'Connor, M., & Woodford, F. P. (1977). *Writing scientific papers in English.* New York: Elsevier.

Ogden, T. E. (1991). *Research proposals: A guide to success.* New York: Raven Press.

Oliu, W. E., Brusaw, C. T., & Alred, G. J. (1984). *Writing that works.* New York: St. Martin's Press.

Olswang, L. B. (1990). Treatment efficacy research: A path to quality assurance. *Asha, 32*(1), 45–47.

O'Shea, H. (1986). Faculty workloads: Myths and realities. *Journal of Nursing Education, 25,* 20–25.

Ottenbacher, K. J. (1990). Clinically relevant designs for rehabilitation research: The idiographic model. *American Journal of Physical Medicine and Rehabilitation, 69*(12), 286–292.

Ottenbacher, K. J. (1991). Statistical conclusion validity: Multiple inferences in rehabilitative research. *American Journal of Physical Medicine and Rehabilitation, 70*(6), 317–322.

Ottenbacher, K. J. (1992). Statistical conclusion validity and type IV errors in rehabilitation research. *American Journal of Physical Medicine and Rehabilitation, 73*(2), 121–125.

Ottenbacher, K. J., & Barrett, K. A. (1990). Statistical conclusion validity of rehabilitation research: A quantitative analysis. *American Journal of Physical Medicine and Rehabilitation, 69*(2), 102–107.

Ownby, R. L. (1987). *Psychological reports.* Brandon, VT: Clinical Psychology Publishing Company.

Paden, E. (1970). *A history of the American Speech and Hearing Association 1925–1958.* Washington, DC: American Speech-Language-Hearing Association.

Pannbacker, M. H., Lass, N. J., & Middleton, G. F. (1988). Making the transition from consumer to producer of research. *Tejas, 14*(1), 33–36.

Pannbacker, M. H., Lass, N. J., & Middleton, G. F. (1993). Ethics education in speech-language pathology and audiology training programs. *Asha, 33*(4), 53–55.

Pannbacker, M. H., & Middleton, G. F. (1991–1992). Common myths about research. *Journal of the National Student Speech-Language-Hearing Association, 19,* 128–137.

Paxson, W. C. (1988). *The mentor guide to writing term papers and reports.* New York: New American Library.

Payne, L., & Anderson, N. (1992). *How to prepare for the NESPA.* San Diego: Singular Publishing Group.

Paynter, E. T., Jordan, W. J., & Finch, D. L. (1990). Patient compliance with cleft palate team regimes. *Journal of Speech and Hearing Disorders, 55*(4), 740–750.

Pecyna, P. M. (1988). Rebus symbol communication training with severely handicapped preschool children: A case study. *Language, Speech and Hearing Services in Schools, 19*(2), 128–143.

Pennebaker, D. F. (1991). Teaching nursing research through collaboration: Costs and benefits. *Journal of Nursing Education, 30*(3), 102–109.

Pezzei, C., & Oratio, A. D. (1991). A multivariate analysis of the job satisfaction of public school speech-language pathologists. *Language, Speech and Hearing Services in Schools, 22*(3), 139–146.

Pfeifer, M. P., & Snodgrass, G. L. (1990). The continued use of retracted invalid scientific literature. *Journal of the American Medical Association, 263*(10), 1420–1423.

Plakke, B. L. (1991). Hearing conservation training of industrial technology teachers. *Language, Speech and Hearing Services in Schools, 22*(3), 134–138.

Plante, E., Kiernan, B., & Betts, J. D. (1994). Research practice method or methodolotry: The qualitative/quantitative debate. *Language, Speech and Hearing Services in Schools, 25*(1), 52–54.

Plante, E., & Vance, R. (1994). Selection of preschool language tests: A data based approach. *Language, Speech and Hearing Services in Schools, 25*(1), 15–24.

Plotnik, A. (1982). *The elements of editing: A modern guide for editors and journalists.* New York: Macmillan.

Polit, D. F., & Hungler, B. P. (1991). *Nursing research: Principles and methods.* Philadelphia: J. B. Lippincott.

Pollock, K. E., & Schwartz, R. G. (1988). Structural aspects of phonological development of a disordered child. *Language, Speech and Hearing Services in Schools, 19*(1), 5–16.

Powell, T. W., Elbert, M., & Dinnsen, D. A. (1991). Stimulability as a factor in the phonological generalization of misarticulating preschool children. *Journal of Speech and Hearing Research, 34*(4), 1318–1328.

Pratt, S. R., Heintzelman, A. T., & Deming, S. E. (1993). The efficacy of using the IBM speech viewer vowel accuracy model to treat young children with hearing impairment. *Journal of Speech and Hearing Research, 36*(4), 1063–1074.

Proctor, A. (1990). Oral language comprehension using hearing aids and tactile aids: Three case studies. *Language, Speech and Hearing Services in Schools, 21*(1), 37–48.

Rao, P., Goldsmith, T., Wilkenson, D., & Hildebrandt, L. (1992). How to keep your customer satisfied: Consumer satisfaction survey. *Hearsay, 7*(11), 34–40, 51.

Ratusnik, D., Klor, B., & Milianti, F. (1979). Institutional research productivity based on publication in the journals of the American Speech and Hearing Association: 1968 through 1977. *Asha, 21,* 99–100.

Read, P. E. (1986). *Foundation fundamentals: A guide for grantseekers* (3rd ed.). New York: The Foundation Center.

Records, N. L., Zomblin, J. B., & Freesa, P. R. (1992). The quality of life of young adults with histories of specific language impairment. *American Journal of Speech-Language Pathology, 1*(2), 45–53.

Redland, A. R. (1989). Mentors and preceptors as models for professional development. *Clinical Nurse Specialist, 3*(2), 70.

Rennie, D. (1990). Editorial peer review in biomedical publications: The first international congress. *Journal of the American Medical Association, 263*(10), 1317.

Rennie, D., & Flanagin, A. (1992). Publication bias: The triumph of hope over experience. *Journal of the American Medical Association, 267*(3), 411–412.

Resnick, D. M. (1993). *Professional ethics for audiologists and speech-language pathologists.* San Diego, CA: Singular Publishing Group.

Rice, M. L., Buhr, J. A., & Oetting, J. B. (1992). Specific language-impaired children's quick incidental learning of words: The effect of a pause. *Journal of Speech and Hearing Research, 35*(4), 1040–1048.

Riegelman, R. (1981). *Studying a study and testing a test: How to read the medical literature.* Boston: Little, Brown.

Ringel, R. (1972). The clinician and the researcher: An artificial dichotomy. *Asha, 14,* 351–353.

Risenberg, D., & Lundberg, G. (1990). The order of authorship: Who's on first. *Journal of the American Medical Association, 264*(14), 1857.

Rockwood, G. Z., & Madison, C. L. (1993). A survey of program selection and expectations of current and prospective graduate students. *National Student Speech-Language-Hearing Association Journal, 20,* 88–98.

Rogers, J. C., Holloway, R. L., & Miller, S. M. (1990). Academic mentoring and family medicine's research productivity. *Family Medicine, 22*(3), 186–190.

Romski, M. A., Joyner, S. E., & Sevcik, R. A. (1987). Vocal communication of a developmentally delayed child: A diary analysis. *Language, Speech and Hearing Services in Schools, 18*(2), 112–130.

Rosenbaum, J., & Rosenbaum, V. (1982). *The writer's survival guide.* Cincinnati, OH: Writer's Digest Books.

Rosenberg, G. G. (1992). Leadership and long-range planning. *Asha, 29*(1), 46–47.

Rosenblum, M. (1989). Principles and practices in searching the scientific literature. In E. P. Woodford (Ed.), *Scientific writing for graduate students.* (pp. 167–178). Bethesda, MD: Council of Biology Editors.

Rosenfeld, R. (1991). Clinical research in otolaryngology journals. *Archives of Otolaryngology: Head and Neck Surgery. 117,* 164–170.

Roth, A. J. (1989). *The research paper.* Belmont, CA: Wadsworth.

Ruscello, D. M., Lass, N. J., French, R. S., & Channel, M. D. (1990). Speech-language pathology students' perception of stutters. *National Student Speech-Language-Hearing Association Journal, 17,* 86–89.

Ruscello, D. M., Lass, N. J., Schmitt, J. F., Pannbacker, M. D., Hoffman, F. M., Miley, M. A., & Robinson, K. L. (1991). Professors' perceptions of stutters. *National Student Speech-Language-Hearing Association Journal, 18,* 142–145.

Ryan, M. N. (1989). Developing and presenting a research poster. *Applied Nursing Research, 2,* 52–55.

St. Louis, K. O., & Durrenberger, C. H. (1993). What communication disorders do experienced clinicians prefer to manage? *Asha, 33*(12), 23–31.

Sands, R. G., Parson, L. A., & Duane, J. (1991). Faculty mentoring in a public university. *Journal of Higher Education, 62,* 174–193.

Saniga, R. D., & Carlin, M. I. (1993). Vocal abuse behaviors in young children. *Language, Speech and Hearing Services in Schools, 24*(2), 79–83.

Sawyer, R., & Stepnick, D. (1989, September). Achieving high quality in slide production for medical education. *ENTechnology,* pp. 32–38.

Schaefer, W. D. (1990). *Education without compromise.* San Francisco, CA: Jossey-Bass.

Schetz, K. F., & Billingsley, B. S. (1992). Speech-language pathologists' perception of administrative support and non-support. *Language, Speech and Hearing Services in Schools, 21*(3), 153–158.

Schiedermayer, D. L., & Siegler, M. (1986). Believing what you read: Responsibilities of medical authors and editors. *Archives of Internal Medicine, 146,* 2043–2044.

Schlip, C. E. (1986). The use of cued speech to correct misarticulation of /s/ and /z/ sounds in an 8-year-old boy with normal hearing. *Language, Speech and Hearing Services in Schools, 17*(4), 270–275.

Schneider, S., & Soto, A. M. (1989). Sexist language: Should we be concerned? *Journal American Women's Medical Association. 44*(3), 79–83.

Schwartz, T. (1988). *Time management for writers.* Cincinnati, OH: Southwestern.

Seal, B. C., & Runyan, S. E. (1988). Time management in clinical supervision: A descriptive study of time allocation. *Asha, 30*(6), 59–61.

Seaton, W. H., & McVey, D. E. (1983). Using SAS for displaying data and preparing poster sessions and materials. *Asha, 25*(5), 41–42.

Seymour, C. M. (1992). Objective: Leadership involvement. *Asha, 29*(5), 45–46.

Seymour, C. M. (1994). Ethical issues. In R. Lubinski & C. Frattali (Eds.), *Professional issues in speech-language pathology and audiology: A textbook* (pp. 61–74). San Diego, CA: Singular Publishing Group.

Sharp, D. (1990). What can and should be done to reduce publication bias? *Journal of the American Medical Association, 263*(10), 1390–1391.

Shaw, H. (1987). *Dictionary of problem words and expressions.* New York: McGraw-Hill.

Shearer, W. S. (1982). *Research procedures in speech, language, and hearing.* Baltimore: Williams & Wilkins.

Shewan, C. M. (1986, November). The survey: An important data collection tool. Miniseminar presented at the annual meeting of the American Speech-Language-Hearing Association, Detroit, MI.

Shewan, C. M. (1988). ASHA women: Education and jobs. *Asha, 25*(6), 39.

Shewan, C. M. (1989, July). ASHA: Plan to showcase research. *Research Bulletin,* pp. 6–19.

Shewan, C. M. (1990a). Plan to showcase research. *Asha, 27*(1), 62–63.

Shewan, C. M. (1990b). *Task force on research proposal for action by ASHA.* Rockville, MD: American Speech-Language-Hearing Association.

Shillig, L. M. (1985, February). The editorial review process: What happens to your manuscript. *Journal of Allied Health,* pp. 149–151.

Shipley, K. G., & McCroskey, R. L. (1978). Strengths and weaknesses in clinical procedures at university clinics. *National Student Speech-Language-Hearing Association Journal, 6*(1), 79–89.

Shore, E. G. (1993). Sanctions and remediation for research misconduct: Differential diagnosis, treatment and prevention. *Academic Medicine, 68*(9)(Suppl.), 544–550.

Shprintzen, R. (1991). Fallibility of clinical research. *Cleft Palate-Craniofacial Journal, 28*(2), 136–140.

Shriberg, L. D., Kwiatkowski, J., & Snyder, T. (1990). Tabletop versus microcomputer assisted speech management: Response evocation phase. *Journal of Speech and Hearing Disorders, 55(4),* 635–655.

Sieber, J. E. (1993). Ethical considerations in planning and conducting research on human subjects. *Academic Medicine, 68(9)(Suppl.),* 59–113.

Siegel, G. M. (1987). The limits of science in communication disorders. *Journal of Speech and Hearing Disorders, 52*(3), 306–312.

Siegel, G. M. (1991–1992). Essential ingredients of a quality MA program in communication disorders: Academic, clinical, research. *National Student Speech-Language-Hearing Association Journal, 19,* 84–88.

Siegel, G. M. (1993). Research: A natural bridge. *Asha, 35*(1), 36–37.

Siegel, G. M., & Ingham, R. J. (1987). Theory and science in communication disorders. *Journal of Speech and Hearing Disorders, 52*(1), 99–104.

Siegel, G. M., & Young, M. A. (1987). Group designs in clinical research. *Journal of Speech and Hearing Disorders, 52*(3), 194–199.

Sigma Xi. (1991). *Honor in science.* Triangle Park, NC: Sigma Xi Scientific Research Society.

Silver, M. A. (1991). Gender differences in career development among psychiatrist administrators. *Journal of the American Medical Women's Association, 46,* 19–22.

Silverman, F. H. (1992). *Legal-ethical considerations, restrictions, and obligations for clinicians who treat communication disorders.* Springfield, IL: Charles C Thomas.

Silverman, F. H. (1993). *Research design and evaluation in speech-language pathology and audiology.* Englewood Cliffs, NJ: Prentice-Hall.

Silverman, F. H., & Marik, J. H. (1993). Teachers' perceptions of stutterers: A replication. *Language, Speech and Hearing Services in Schools, 24*(2), 108.

Silverstein, B., Fisher, W. P., Kilgore, K. M., Harley, J. P., & Harvey, R. F. (1992). Applying psychometric criteria to functional assessment in medical rehabilitation: II. Defining interval measures. *Archives of Physical Medicine Rehabilitation, 73,* 507–518.

Simmonds, D. (1984). How to produce a good poster. *Medical Teacher, 6*(1), 10–13.

Slater, S. C. (1992). Portrait of the professions. *Asha, 29*(7), 61–65.

Slater, S. C. (1993). Mentoring: An enriching experience. *Asha, 30*(4), 55.

Smith, J., Carter, M., & Gilder, G. (1988). Trends in time allocation for school speech-language pathologists: A need for change. *Hearsay, 3,* 24–26.

Sorrels, B. D. (1983). *The nonsexist communicator.* Englewood Cliffs, NJ: Prentice-Hall.

Sparks, R. D. (1989). Matching ideas and funds. *Asha, 31,* 77, 99.

Spradley, J. P. (1979). *The ethnographic interview.* New York: Holt, Rinehart & Winston.

Stager, S. V., & Ludlow, C. L. (1993). Speech production changes under fluency-evoking conditions in nonstuttering speakers. *Journal of Speech and Hearing Research, 36*(2), 245–253.

Stainback, S., & Stainback, W. (1988). *Understanding and conducting qualitative research.* Reston, VA: Council for Exceptional Children.

Steckler, A., McLeroy, K. L., Goodman, R. M., Bird, S. T., & McCormick, L. (1992). Toward integrating qualitative and quantitative methods: An introduction. *Health Education Quarterly, 19*(1), 108.

Stephens, I. (1991). Mentor-mentee: A satisfying process. *Communicologist, 16,* 3, 10.

Sternberg, D. (1981). *How to complete and survive a doctoral dissertation.* New York: St. Martin's Press.

Stevens, J. P. (1991). On seeing the statistician, and some analysis caveats. *American Journal of Physical Medicine and Rehabilitation, 70,* S151–S152.

Stewart, B. A. (1992). Objective: Leadership involvement. *Asha, 29*(5), 45–46.

Stouffer, J. L., & Tyler, R. S. (1990). Characterization of tinnitus by tinnitus patients. *Journal of Speech and Hearing Disorders, 55*(3), 439–453.

Strange, K., & Hekelman, F. (1990). Mentoring needs and family medicine faculty. *Family Medicine, 22,* 183–185.

Strunk, W., & White, E. B. (1979). *The elements of style.* New York: Macmillan.

Sturner, R. A., Layton, T. L., Evans, A. W., Heller, J. H., Funk, S. G., & Machas, M. W. (1994). Preschool speech and language screening: A review of currently available tests. *American Journal of Speech Language Pathology, 3*(1), 25–36.

Tawney, J. W., & Gast, D. L. (1984). *Single subject research in special education.* Columbus, OH: Charles E. Merrill.

Teitelbaum, H. (1989). *How to write a thesis.* New York: Arco.

Thal, D., & Tobias, S. (1994). Relationship between language and gesture in normally developing and late-talking toddlers. *Journal of Speech and Hearing Research, 37*(1), 157–170.

Theil, C. M. (1992). Developing a comprehensive, manageable quality improvement program. *Hearsay, 7*(1), 28–33.

Thomas, J. P., & Lawrence, T. S. (1990). Common deficiencies on NIDRR research applications. *American Journal of Physical Medicine and Rehabilitation, 69*(2), 73–76.

Tibbits, D. F. (1992). Objective: Leadership involvement. *Asha, 29*(5), 45–46.

Towne, R. L., & Entwisle, L. M. (1993). Metaphonic comprehension in adolescents with traumatic brain injury and in adolescents with language learning disability. *Language, Speech and Hearing Services in Schools, 24*(2), 100–107.

Travers, B. (1983). Improving speech and language services through effective time management. *Language, Speech and Hearing Services in Schools, 14,* 86–91.

Troyka, L. Q. (1990). *Simon and Schuster handbook for writers.* Englewood Cliffs, NJ: Prentice-Hall.

Trudeau, M. D., & Crowe, B. J. (1988). Voice disorders: Searching for needles of wisdom in a haystack of journals. *Asha, 30*(5), 35–37.

U.S. Department of Health and Human Services. (1993). *NIH guide for grants and contracts.* Bethesda, MD: National Institutes of Health.

University of Chicago. (1982). *The Chicago manual of style.* Chicago: The University of Chicago Press.

Vafadar, A. C., & Utt, H. A. (1993). A survey of speech-language pathologists' attitudes about self-perceived knowledge of, and competency in dealing with social dialects: Language differences versus language disorders. *National Student Speech-Language-Hearing Association Journal, 20,* 65–72.

Van der Lely, H. K. J., & Howard, D. (1993). Children with specific language impairment: Linguistic impairment or short-term memory deficit? *Journal of Speech and Hearing Research, 36*(6), 1193–1207.

Van Tasell, D. J. (1993). Hearing loss, speech, and hearing aids. *Journal of Speech and Hearing Research, 36*(2), 228–244.

Venn, M. L., Wolert, M., Fleming, L. A., DeCesare, L. D., Morris, A., & Cuffs, M. S. (1993). Effects of teaching pre-school peers to use the mand-model procedure during snack activities. *American Journal of Speech-Language Pathology, 2*(1), 38–46.

Venolia, J. (1987). *Rewrite right.* Berkeley, CA: Ten Speed Press/ Periwinkle Press.

Ventry, I., & Schiavetti, N. (1986). *Evaluating research in speech pathology and audiology.* New York: Macmillan.

Vetter, D. K. (1985). Evaluation of clinical intervention: Accountability. *Seminars in Speech and Language, 6*(1), 55–65.

Violette, J., & Swisher, L. (1992). Echolalic responses by a child with autism to four experimental conditions of sociolinguistic input. *Journal of Speech and Hearing Research, 35*(1), 139–147.

Waltz, C., Nelson, B., & Chambers, S. (1985). Assigning publication credits. *Nursing Outlook, 33*(5), 233–238.

Warren, R. L. (1986). Research design: Considerations for the clinician. In R. Chapey (Ed.), *Language intervention strategies in adult aphasia* (pp. 66–79). Baltimore: Williams & Wilkins.

Warren, S. F., Yoder, P. J., Gazdag, G. E., Kin, K., & Jones, H. A. (1993). Facilitating prelinguistic communication skills in young children with developmental delay. *Journal of Speech and Hearing Research, 36*(1), 83–97.

Webster, D., & Conrad, C. (1986). Using faculty research performance for academic quality rankings. *New Directions for Institutional Research, 50,* 43–57.

Weidenborner, S., & Caruso, D. (1982). *Writing research papers.* New York: St. Martin's Press.

Weiner, I. S., & Eisen, R. G. (1985). Clinical research: The case study and single subject designs. *Journal of Allied Health, 14,* 191–201.

Weismer, S. E., Murray-Branch, J., & Miller, J. F. (1993). Comparison of two methods for promoting productive vocabulary in late talkers. *Journal of Speech and Hearing Research, 36*(4), 1037–1050.

Welsh, R., & Slater, S. (1993). The state of infant hearing identification programs. *Asha, 33*(4), 49–52.

White, J. F. (1988). The perceived role of mentoring in the career development and success of academic nurse-administrators. *Journal of Professional Nursing, 4*, 178–179.

White, V. (Ed.). (1983). *Grant proposals that succeeded.* New York: Plenum Press.

Whurr, R., Lorch, M. P., & Nye, C. (1992). A meta-analysis of studies carried out between 1946 and 1988 concerned with the efficacy of speech and language therapy treatment for aphasic patients. *European Journal of Disorders of Communication, 27*(1), 1–17.

Williams, A. L. (1991). Generalization patterns associated with training least phonological knowledge. *Journal of Speech and Hearing Research, 34*(3), 722–733.

Williams, R., & Blackburn, R. T. (1988). Mentoring and junior faculty productivity. *Journal of Nursing Education, 27*, 204–209.

Wilson, K. S., Blackman, R. C., Hall, R. E., & Eichultz, G. E. (1991). Motives of language assessment: A survey of California public school clinicians. *Language, Speech and Hearing Services in Schools, 22*(4), 236–241.

Windsor, J., Doyle, S. S., & Siegel, G. M. (1994). Language acquisition after mutism: A longitudinal case study of autism. *Journal of Speech and Hearing Research, 37*(1), 96–105.

Wing, C. S. (1990). Defective infant formulas and expressive language problems: A case study. *Language, Speech, and Hearing Services in Schools, 21*(1), 22–27.

Wofford, M., Boysen, A., & Riding, L. (1991). A research mentoring process. *Asha, 31*(9), 39–42.

Wolery, M., Venn, M. L., Schroeder, C., Holcombe, A., Huffnay, K., Marlin, C. G., Brookfield, J., & Fleming, L. A. (1994). A survey of the extent to which speech-language pathologists are employed in preschool programs. *Language, Speech and Hearing Services in Schools, 25*(1), 2–8.

Woodford, F. P. (1967). Sounder thinking through clearer writing. *Science, 156*, 743–745.

Woodford, F. P. (Ed.). (1989a). *Scientific writing for graduate students.* Bethesda, MD: Council of Biology Editors.

Woodford, F. P. (1989b). Writing a journal article. In F. P. Woodford (Ed.), *Scientific writing for graduate students* (pp. 3–114). Bethesda, MD: Council of Biology Editors.

Woodward, C. A. (1988). Questionnaire construction and question writing for research in medical education. *Medical Education, 22*, 347–363.

Woolf, P. (1986). Pressure to publish and fraud in science. *Annals of Internal Medicine, 104*(12), 254–256.

Wylie, N. R., & Fuller, J. W. (1985). Enhancing faculty vitality through collaboration among colleagues. In R. G. Baldwin (Ed.), *Incentives for faculty vitality*. New directions for higher education (pp. 99–110). San Francisco: Jossey-Bass.

Yairi, E., & Carrico, D. M. (1992). Early childhood stuttering: Pediatricians' attitudes and practices. *American Journal of Speech-Language Pathology, 1*(3), 55–62.

Yale University School of Medicine. (1987). Creating poster sessions. *MG & P* (The Department of Medical Graphics and Photography), *4,* 1–4.

Yoder, P. J., Kaiser, A. P., Alpert, C., & Fischer, R. (1993). Following the child's lead when teaching nouns to pre-schoolers with mental retardation. *Journal of Speech and Hearing Research, 36*(1), 158–167.

Young, A. (1986). *The manager's handbook*. New York: Crown Publishers.

Young, M. A. (1993). Supplementing tests of statistical significance: Variation accounted for. *Journal of Speech and Hearing Research, 36*(3), 644–656.

Zinsser, W. (1988). *On writing well*. New York: Harper & Row.

GLOSSARY

Abstract: brief description of a paper usually located at the beginning of an article.

Alpha level: a level of significance.

Analysis: the process of organizing data so that research questions can be answered.

Analysis of variance: a parametric statistical procedure for simultaneously comparing three or more means; also known as ANOVA.

Analytic induction: an approach for analyzing qualitative data by alternating back and forth between tentative explanation for each repetition and gradual refinement of emerging hypothesis.

Applied research: research that seeks to answer practical questions such as those pertaining to prevention and management of communication disorders.

Asymmetrical distribution: a distribution of values that is not symmetrical. Also known as skewed.

Attrition: loss of subject(s) during the course of a study.

Bar graph: *see* Histogram.

Baseline measure: measurement of dependent variable before experimental intervention.

Basic research: research that is often theoretical; designed to seek answers that explain and/or predict phenomena.

Between-subject design: design that uses two groups of subjects, each group assigned to a different level of the independent variable.

Bias: result of any systematic occurrence which results in a sample that in some way is not representative of the population.

Bimodal distribution: a distribution that has two peaks.

Bivariate (statistical) tests: test used to analyze significance of the relationship between two variables simultaneously.

Blind review: review of a manuscript so that neither author nor reviewer is identifiable to the other.

Call for papers: a request to submit proposals for presentation at convention or meeting.

Case study: intensive study of an individual, group, institution, or community.

Casual relationship: relationship between two variables so that presence or absence of one variable (cause) determines presence, absence, or value of the other (effect).

Categorical variable: a variable with discrete values.

Central tendency: measures representing the average or typical score in a distribution (mean, median, mode).

Clinical research: research designed to generate knowledge to guide clinical practice in speech-language pathology and audiology; also known as applied research.

Confidence interval: an inferential statistic for estimating range of values within which a population parameter lies.

Confidence level: estimated probability that a population value lies within a given confidence interval.

Construct validity: the extent to which a test or questionnaire measures what it is supposed to measure.

Consumer: an individual who critically reviews research and attempts to use and apply research in clinical practice in speech-language pathology and audiology.

Content analysis: a systematic, objective method for quantifying content of qualitative data in diaries, interviews, articles, speeches, and so on.

Content validity: a logical examination of all behaviors that need to be measured in order to adequately answer the question.

Continuous variable: a variable that can be expressed in any numerical value including fractions to represent a large range of values along a continuum.

Contract: a written agreement signed by participants (contractor and contractee) outlining terms and conditions.

Control group: a group that does not receive treatment; equivalent to the experimental group in age, sex, and so on.

Copyright: exclusive right to produce and sell copies of an author's work for a specified time period.

Correlation: tendency for variation in one variable to be related to variation in another variable; an interrelation between two or more variables.

Correlation coefficient: a statistic that describes the strength and direction of relationship between two variables.

Correlational research: research designed to explore relationships among variables of interest without active intervention.

Cost-benefit analysis: an evaluation comparing financial costs with financial gains attributed to a program or intervention.

Criterion-related (predictive) validity. the measure of an attribute to predict future performance.

Cross sectional: a comparison of behaviors or characteristics of subjects from various age groups.

Data: numerical or descriptive quantities that define the concept being studied; singular is datum.

Database: information accessed by using electronic hardware.

Dependent variable: variable that is the effect of unknown etiology(ies) and must be described in operational terms.

Descriptive research: studies that use a nonstatistical method of organizing raw data for clarity in communication and interpretation.

Descriptive statistics: procedures for describing and analyzing quantitative data.

Design: the structure of a study organized for the purpose of revealing cause-and-effect relationships by controlling variables, comparing groups, or analyzing specific characteristics of individuals or groups.

Direct costs: expenses related to personnel, fringe benefits, travel, equipment, and supplies.

Dissertation: a long, scholarly paper written by a candidate for a doctoral degree.

Distribution: form or shape of numerical values in a sample.

Double speak: confusing terminology.

Draft: unrevised, working manuscript; several usually are needed.

Duplicate submission: submission of the same manuscript to two or more different journals; violation of ethical conduct.

Empirical evidence: objective evidence gathered through the scientific approach.

Error of measurement: measure of the degree of deviation between true scores and obtained scores.

Evaluation research: research involving the collection and analysis of information related to effects of a program, policy, or procedure.

Experimental research: research in which the independent variable is controlled in order to measure its effect on the dependent variables.

Ex post facto research: research conducted after variations in the independent variable have occurred; retrospective study.

Field research: in-depth research of individuals or groups conducted in naturalistic settings.

Figure: any type of illustration other than a table.

Foundation: a nongovernment, nonprofit organization with funds and activities managed by its own trustees or board of directors.

Fragmented publication: *see* least publishable unit.

Fraud: major unethical conduct; violation of three or more of the four norms of science: universalism, communality, disinterestedness, organized skepticism.

Frequency distribution: an organization of numerical values from lowest to highest, on the x-axis together with a count of the number of times each value occurred on the y-axis.

Frequency polygon: graphic display of a frequency distribution; created by drawing straight lines between the successive midpoints of class intervals.

Generalizability: the extent to which findings are representative of the entire population.

Gift authorship: unjustified authorship.

Grant: an award of financial support.

Grant management: responsibility for activities and expenditures associated with management of a project funded by a grant.

Grant proposal: formal application for a grant; includes introduction, problem statement or needs assessment, objectives, method, and budget.

Grantsmanship: the knowledge and skills needed to secure financial support.

Graphic output: visual display of data in graphic form such as a scattergram.

Grounded theory: an approach for analyzing qualitative data through constant comparison to develop and refine categories; theoretical concepts are discovered in the data.

Group designs: design involving comparison of average or typical performance of a group to other groups or conditions.

Handout: a written supplement to an oral or poster presentation.

Hawthorne effect: an effect on the dependent variable caused by changes in behavior that occur because subjects know they are participating in a study.

Histogram: graphic display of frequency distribution data in which scores (often in group intervals) are plotted on the x-axis and frequency (or percent of cases) is plotted on the y-axis. Also known as bar graph.

Historical research: library research to establish facts and relationships about past events.

Honorary authorship: unjustified authorship.

Hypothesis: statement concerning relationship between variables; formulated to test theories.

Incomplete authorship: failure to include individuals who contributed substantially to a project.

Independent variable: variable with known qualities which explains the dependent variable; may be manipulated to determine effect on dependent variable.

Indirect costs: costs such as heating/cooling, electricity, maintenance, security, administrative costs.

Inferential statistics: statistics used to test hypotheses by drawing inferences or generalizations from small groups to larger groups.

Institutional Review Board (IRB): a group of individuals who review research proposals relative to ethical considerations.

Intervention: experimental treatment or manipulation in experimental research. *See* Manipulation.

Irresponsible authorship: problems related to unjustified authorship, incomplete authorship, and/or inaccurate quotations and/or references.

Kurtosis: flatness or peakedness of a graphed distribution.

Lazy writing: closely related to plagiarism except that references are cited.

Least publishable unit (LPU): reporting same study in installments; same as fragmented publication.

Leptokurtic: sharply peaked graphed distribution with a short tail.

Level of significance: significance level selected to reject the null hypothesis established before statistical analysis to reduce the risk of making a Type I or Type II error.

Literature review: critical review of literature to identify weaknesses and strengths of prior studies, and identify research needs.

Longitudinal: the same group of subjects is followed over time.

Mañana syndrome: procrastination; frequently results in missing deadlines.

Manipulation: intervention or treatment in an experimental or quasi-experimental study; the independent variable is manipulated to assess its impact on the dependent variable. *See also* Intervention.

Manuscript: an unpublished paper.

Mean: simple arithmetic average.

Measurement: the assignment of numbers to objects according to rules to characterize quantities of some attribute.

Median: a statistic describing the central tendency of scores in an ordinal scale; the midpoint in a set of values (same number of values above as below the median).

Mentee: an individual seeking guidance in a particular area from one or more persons experienced in that area of study or activity.

Mentor: an individual with specific expertise who provides support and guidance to an individual with less experience.

Meta-analysis: a technique for quantitatively combining results of several studies on a given topic.

Mixed group design: combines within-subjects and between-subjects designs to investigate effects of treatment for which carryover effects would be a problem while repeatedly sampling the behavior.

Modality: number of peaks in a graphed distribution.

Modality of distribution: number of peaks in the graphic display of numerical values; unimodal, multimodal (often bimodal).

Mode: the most frequently occurring value in a distribution.

Multimodal: two or more peaks or high points evident in a graphed distribution.

Multivariate tests: statistical procedures used to study the relationship among three or more variables.

Needs assessment: data collected to estimate needs of a group, community, or organization.

Negative relationship: a relationship between two variables in which there is a tendency for higher values of one variable to be associated with lower values of the other.

Negatively skewed distribution: an asymmetrical distribution in which there is a disproportionally high number of high values.

Nonexperimental research: descriptive (nonstatistical) organization of data; or ex post facto research.

Nonparametric statistics: a type of inferential statistics that does not involve vigorous assumptions about the parameters of the population from which the sample was drawn; used for nominal and ordinal measures.

Normal distribution: symmetrical graphic display of the numerical values.

Null hypothesis: statement that there is no relationship between variables under study.

On line: data that are accessed by the user who interacts directly with the electronic program to retrieve desired information.

Outliers: wild atypical numerical values.

Parametric statistics: a type of inferential statistics that involves making assumptions about the parameters of the population from which the research sample was drawn; used for interval measures.

Patchwork plagiarism: a verbatim quote with single words changed; uncited references. Less severe form of plagiarism.

Peer reviewers: individuals who review, critique and make recommendations about research reports or proposals.

Pilot study: a preliminary study designed to determine advisability for further study or call attention to research possibilities.

Plagiarism: thievery of style, ideas, or phrases. Ranges from word-for-word (exact) to patchwork (some words changed); frequently related to lack of proper referencing.

Platykurtic: a flat distribution with long tail.

Population: the group the research question refers to.

Positive relationship: a relationship between two variables in which there is a tendency for high values of one variable to be associated with high values of the other.

Positively skewed distribution: an asymmetrical graphic distribution in which there is a disproportionally high number of low values.

Poster presentation: a visual display summarizing research presented on vertical bulletin boards.

Power: the probability of a statistical test to reject the null hypothesis when it is in fact false.

Principle investigator: the individual who formulates research questions, designs the project, obtains funding, manages the project, oversees data analysis and preparation of the project for publication.

Procrastination: needless delay possibly causing discomfort, anxiety, "busyness," or binging.

Professional jargon: terminology peculiar to a specific profession.

Proposal: document describing what will be stated, specific research problem, its significance, planned procedures, and when funding is required, the cost of the research.

Qualitative research: research designed to investigate real-life events or situations without reference to hypothesis or theory, allowing researcher's subjective point of view; also known as field research, hermeneutic, naturalistic inquiry, phenomenological research, symbolic interactionism, descriptive research, interpretive research, and ethnographic study.

Quantitative research: research that generates data capable of being organized in graphs and descriptive statistical forms.

Quartiles: range of values within the first quarter ($\frac{1}{4}$), second quarter, third quarter, and fourth quarter of the data.

Quasi-experimental research: research involving manipulation of an independent variable without a comparison group or the randomization of subjects into groups.

Quasi-statistics: a means of analyzing qualitative data by tabulating frequency of occurrences.

Randomization: a method of selecting subjects that ensures that everyone in the population has an equal chance of being included in the study.

Range: distance between the lowest and highest values in a distribution.

Raw data: unorganized data, can be numerical or verbal descriptions.

Redundant publication: practice of reporting the same study more than once; also known as self-plagiarism.

Relationship: connection between or among two or more variables.

Reliability: repeatability, consistency among repeated measures or observations.

Replicate: repeat; duplicate.

Request for Application (RFA): a solicited proposal announcement.

Request for Proposal (RFP): a solicited proposal announcement.

Response rate: rate of participation in a survey, calculated by dividing the number of persons participating by the number of persons sampled.

Sampling: procedures for selecting the portion of a population to serve as subjects for a study.

Scales of measurement: a means of assigning numbers to events or objects according to prescribed rules.

Scatter plot: a graphic display of the relationship between two variables; also known as scatter diagram or scattergram.

Secondary analysis: a study of previously gathered data.

Self-plagiarism: reporting the same study more than once. Also known as redundant publication.

Semi-interquartile range: range of values between the first value of the second quartile and the last value of the third quartile.

Semi-longitudinal: combination of cross-sectional and longitudinal approaches; selecting subjects at the low end of designated age spans and following them until they reach upper limits of that age span.

Single subject design: a research design that provides controlled conditions in which to determine the performance of one or a few subjects to establish cause-and-effect relations (i.e. make conclusions concerning the effects of treatment on behavior).

Skewed distribution: an asymmetrical graphic display of numerical values; may be positively (longer tail points to right) or negatively skewed (longer tail points to left).

Solicited proposal: an invited proposal with a specific deadline; usually accompanied by RFA or RFP.

Standard deviation: a variability measure of the degree to which each value deviates from the mean; abbreviated SD or small Greek (σ).

Standard error of measurement (SEM): estimate of the standard deviation of a population based on the distribution from a sample group from that population.

Subjects: individuals selected to participate in a study because they possess the same characteristics as the population they represent.

Survey research: data are collected by asking people for information.

Table: an illustration that displays data in tabular form. Not a figure.

Tenure: institutional commitment to continuous employment of faculty.

Test-retest reliability: how well subjects perform on one set of measurements as compared to their performance on a second evaluation of the same measurements.

Thesis: a paper written by a candidate for the master's degree.

Thesis option: academic program in which a thesis is optional (i.e., not required).

Trimodal: three peaks or high points in a graphic distribution.

Two-tailed test: test of a hypothesis using both ends of the distribution to determine a range of improbable values.

Type I error: incorrectly rejecting the null hypothesis.

Type II error: incorrectly accepting the null hypothesis.

Unethical: failure to adhere to ethical guidelines.

Unimodal: one peak or high point in a graphic distribution.

Unjustified authorship: authors who did not make substantial contribution.

Unsolicited proposal: proposal for which there is no specific deadline for submission; usually accepted and reviewed at any time.

Validity: appropriateness of information gathered to accurately answer a specific question.

Vanity publisher: a publisher that requires authors to pay for publication.

Variability: spread or dispersion of the data.

Variable: a trait capable of change or modification.

Within-subject designs: a design in which every subject is exposed to all of the experimental conditions.

Appendix

131 Suggestions and Observations on Reporting the Results of Research

1. Never give up on any writing project.
2. Admit your mistakes; don't be afraid to say "I made a mistake."
3. Remember that editors are not biased.
4. Demand excellence and be willing to work for it.
5. Avoid biased comments.
6. Remember that the most important thing is intellectual integrity.
7. Choose your co-authors carefully; begin this process early.
8. Attend writing seminars.
9. Join a journal club.
10. Never cheat.
11. Never argue with an editor.
12. Learn to identify your strengths and weaknesses.
13. Resist the temptation to criticize others.
14. Read an article in a scholarly journal every day.
15. Learn to write in small blocks of time.
16. Submit written projects on time.
17. Do not be afraid to rewrite.
18. Strive for excellence, not perfection.
19. Get acquainted with a published author.
20. Keep your desk and work area neat.

21. Do not waste time responding to your critics.
22. Avoid negative people.
23. Resist telling people about your publication victories.
24. Share your defeats as well as your victories.
25. Be suspicious of all published literature.
26. Never take action when you are angry.
27. Do battle against bias whenever your find it.
28. Be curious.
29. Return borrowed books and materials.
30. Choose publication projects that are of interest to you.
31. Do not waste time grieving over past projects; learn from them and move on.
32. Resist giving advice about publishing unless asked.
33. Keep deadlines.
34. Editors and reviewers are trained to identify weaknesses not strengths.
35. Avoid plagiarism like the plague.
36. Maintain a positive attitude.
37. Discipline yourself to manage time wisely.
38. Accept failure as part of publishing.
39. Take a nap on Sunday afternoons.
40. Compliment others' publication efforts.
41. Learn to disagree without being disagreeable.
42. Be tactful, never purposefully alienate anyone.
43. Never underestimate the power of hard work.
44. Do not say you do not have enough time; make the time.
45. Do not delay acting on a good idea.
46. Be wary of people who tell you about their publishing expertise.
47. Remember that productive writers do what unproductive writers do not want to do.
48. Substitute the word *opportunity* for the word *problem.*
49. If something sounds too easy, it probably is.
50. Own a good reference and style manual.
51. Remember no one makes it alone; acknowledge those who help you.
52. Be a self-starter.
53. Reward even small successes.
54. Maintain a positive attitude.
55. Learn how to use a computer; it saves time and effort.
56. Do not procrastinate.
57. Prioritize your schedule.
58. Share the credit.
59. Do more than is expected.

60. Select a co-author your own age so that you can grow old together.
61. Every person you meet knows something you do not; learn from them.
62. Do it right the first time.
63. Be human: Do not be afraid to say "I don't know."
64. Be human: Do not be afraid to say "I need help."
65. Never compromise your integrity.
66. Show respect for others' publications, regardless of how trivial they may seem.
67. Do not use time or words carelessly.
68. Get organized.
69. Be open to new ideas.
70. Set goals.
71. Respond promptly to "Calls for Papers" and requests for revision.
72. Keep several writing projects going simultaneously.
73. Become someone's mentor.
74. Do not be afraid to fail.
75. Do not opinionate.
76. Use the third person.
77. Do not be taken in by nonproductive writers.
78. Write a "letter to the editor" of a scholarly journal.
79. Regularly review the professional literature.
80. Never accept honorary authorship.
81. Respond to reprint requests promptly.
82. Accept criticism gracefully.
83. Find a mentor.
84. Cover your keyboard when leaving your computer unattended in the same room with a cat who enjoys "revising" your work.
85. Keep it simple.
86. Write on a daily basis.
87. Know where to look.
88. Know the similarities between clinical and research activities.
89. Do not publish for the wrong reason(s).
90. Maintain high ethical standards.
91. Know the difference between good and bad publications.
92. Develop a research support system.
93. Be careful in selecting a publication advisor.
94. Avoid blocking.
95. Have a good supply of printer ribbons on hand.
96. Give research a high priority.

97. Know the joys of publishing.
98. Know that those who criticize most usually publish least, if at all.
99. Be aware that those who do not want to play the publication game usually do not know how to play the game.
100. Remember an unfinished written project is one that someone gave up on.
101. Do good writing.
102. Tackle important written projects.
103. Do not attack others' publications.
104. Write clearly.
105. Use reviewers' comments constructively.
106. Be aware of publication fads and trends.
107. Return library books on time.
108. Exercise and eat healthy.
109. Give yourself daily "quiet time" to think.
110. Never laugh at anyone's research.
111. Never apologize for being early for submitting a paper.
112. Read the articles nominated each year for ASHA Awards.
113. Keep a log of your research and writing efforts.
114. Seize every opportunity for additional research training.
115. When your manuscript is rejected, don't lose the lesson.
116. Read a book about research.
117. Take the stairs when it's five flights or less.
118. When it comes to revising a paper, know when to stop.
119. Deadlines are important. Meet them.
120. Select a research partner who's strong where you are weak.
121. Accept the fact that, regardless of how many papers you publish, you will sometimes be rejected.
122. Never miss an opportunity to go to the library or read a professional journal.
123. Hold yourself to the highest ethical standards.
124. Remember that how you write something is as important as what you write.
125. Publish your research; it is a way to achieve immortality.
126. Spend your time and effort creating not criticizing.
127. Encourage anyone who is trying to do research.
128. Choose a research partner the way you choose a bridge or diving partner. Select someone who is strong where you are weak.
129. Approach research with reckless abandon.
130. Publication is a privilege, not simply a right.
131. Select a research partner who can find what you have lost.

INDEX